MIND HACKING SECRETS

21 NEUROSCIENCE WAYS TO DEVELOP FAST, CLEAR &
CRITICAL THINKING. LEARN HOW TO TRAIN YOUR
BRAIN TO THINK FASTER AND CLEARLY IN 2 WEEKS.

SCOTT SHARP

CONTENTS

Do you long to be able to have clear thinking, a clear mind, organizational skills, and the ability to recall information more efficiently? Are there moments when you wish you could learn faster, remember more, and be more productive?

There are methods that you will be able to use to keep your brain sharp through critical thinking, improved decision-making skills, and problem-solving abilities.

This book is going to be a practical guide for you to improve the way that you think overall. What matters most is the bulk of the reading, which will include the important "how" of this process. We are going to teach you how you can use your brain to its fullest potential. There will be a focus on practice and precise methods to develop fast, critical, and clear thinking.

The purpose of this reading will be to provide you with foundational "how-to" knowledge so you can apply what you learn to your life to see instant results. Your problem now is that you are unsatisfied with your mind. We have the solution, and so do you! We will provide you with all that is needed to unlock the secrets of your mind. This is a must-read for anyone that wants to know how they can get the things they desire most with the full use of their brain. It is our promise that you will discover all that you need within the world of neuroscience inside this book. The longer you wait to start to train your brain, the harder it becomes to alter your methods of thinking. Don't put this off anymore! Start to find the tools needed for a happier and healthier mind before it is too late!

The solution to your biggest neuroscience issues lies within your brain. We are going to give you actionable steps to help you get the results you want. We will teach you how to think fast, clearly, and critically. We will help you improve your focus, reasoning, judgment, analysis, and ability to make certain choices. We will help you increase your writing skills, as well as your ability to speak. We will make it easier to remember more, think and learn faster, and use certain neuroscience methods to understand better how your brain works the way that it does.

There is no pill, surgery, or another quick method that is going to give you a new way of thinking. All the changes that you wish to make within your neurology are entirely possible by using your brain!

The brain that we have is the only one that we will ever experience. However, this doesn't mean that we can't alter the way in which we think. The experiences that we lived through, the moments that built our life, and the cherished times that we remember all play a massive role in forming the people that we are today.

We are going to help you discover the methods with which you can think faster under pressure. There are many stressful experiences that we will go through within our lives that make it difficult to know what the right choice is. Sometimes you might feel pressure from others, but there are plenty of instances of feeling that pressure within ourselves that can make it hard to know what the right decision for our future might be.

Our brain is a strong organ that we rarely use to the fullest potential. We already have the tools within us to optimize the efficiency of this brain. It all starts by knowing how to think accurately and analyzing the situations that are presented to us.

How frequently do you feel as though you have been fooled? Are there certain mistakes or mental traps that you wish you could remove yourself from? Whether it is a manipulative family member or the influential media that is making you feel this way, you are strong enough to break free from these mental restrictions that keep you trapped within a toxic cycle of thinking.

What many of us desire more than anything is the ability to

have better focus and concentration. How many times have you found yourself in a troubling position because you couldn't remember what someone told you, or perhaps you struggled to remember certain parts of important information? Maybe you couldn't recall something that you went through, or you forgot an important detail. You can train your brain to think with focus and increase your concentration levels to prevent you from forgetting the same things over and over again.

It is highly suggested that you have a notebook or journal to write things down in as we go through this book. Research shows that when you focus on writing things down, it helps you to remember better. Whenever we have a strategy, routine, or exercise for you to do, take note of this. You will learn throughout this three-part book the methods, strategies, and practical ways to increase your mental abilities. At the end of the book, we have 21 quick tips for you to take note of and apply to your daily life in real ways that are achievable. Stay open-minded and dedicated to learning throughout this process, and you will discover all that you have wished you could gain in this life!

[PART 1]
THINK CLEAR

[1]

BEST WAYS AND STRATEGIES TO DEVELOP CLEAR THINKING

You weren't just born with the brain that you have now. We were essentially born with a blank slate, though some genetics helped shape our brain. However, the experiences that you have gone through, the things you've learned, and the lessons that were hardest to swallow all played a very crucial role in building the person that you are today. Though it sometimes feels as though you try very hard and see little results in terms of overall brainpower gain, it is entirely possible to shape the way you think for a happier and healthier life.

Studies show that stress is one of the main reasons that we have trouble thinking clearly. As you can already start to gather, clear thinking doesn't happen when we only focus on the patterns of thought we have. Everything that we do in our life can contribute to the mental cloudiness that makes even the smallest tasks a challenge. It is crucial that we give ourselves the chance to think clearly so that we can better understand ourselves and what we want from this life.

Studies have shown that stress can even change the shape of our brain! What your childhood was like, the school you went to, the friends and family you have in your life, and so much more all contribute to the way that you operate. Stress is natural but can be a heightened response depending on a number of factors. Even though your brain might have been shaped to be a certain way now, you have all the power you will ever need to turn that around and create a healthy brain that functions optimally.

Creating Purpose and Finding Meaning

You have to understand first what it is that gets in the way of your clearer thinking. What is it that keeps you from thinking properly? Which thoughts are clouding your mind? Do you frequently have distractions around you that make it almost impossible to properly function?

If you want to be able to reduce your distractions and focus on what's most important in life, you have to know what's important. If you don't have your strong goals and virtues, then it is going to be nearly impossible to understand what's important. Often, we create a life around expectations. Maybe getting a job, finding a spouse, and having children seem important to you, but this isn't your main passion.

This is because those initial desires are things that we are taught to want to have. Create your goals and you will be happier than trying to please someone else's.

We have to be in charge of our future, our intentions. Having healthy goals is going to be another part of this. You have to set your own goals. Others might inspire you to think of some, and you can discover certain things you want by talking to other people. However, if you don't know how to create your purpose, you will be miserable throughout your life!

Allow yourself to be yourself. Above all else, you have to be the person that you were meant to be. If you feel like you are sacrificing part of yourself, then you are not staying true to your character. Let's take a look at some strategies to help you discover what your true purpose and meaning in this world might be.

Ask yourself which challenges you are comfortable with. Is there anything that you don't mind doing that other people dread being a part of? Have you come face to face with a challenge that wasn't that hard to get over that other people in the world might never be able to complete?

Truly think about what you would do if you found out you were going to die within a year. What would you wish you had thought more about? Which areas of your cognition would you be fine with ignoring? What would you be fine with forgetting for the rest of your life? A year ahead is a good time period because you might not even be able to afford to quit your job right away! Rather than thinking, "I'm going to quit my job and explore the world," you can come up with a practical way to make it through the biggest challenges.

Create your own virtue. It is good to have a moral standing that is common with others. This might be a religion, for example. However, you can't only follow the rules that were created for you. You have to come up with your beliefs and discover the things that are most important to you. If you don't believe in the things that you live by, then you won't be able to create true virtue and meaning.

Already, as you start to confront your thinking abilities, you have the chance to find clarity and increase cognition. When you learn to focus on the things that are important and forget the things that don't matter, you generally enjoy life more. Strip your life down to the very core. When you go to bed at night and are alone with your thoughts, who are you really? When you have nothing to do but sit outside with nature, which parts of life do you think about? Who do you want right by your side?

If you don't have this, then you are not going to be able to find benefits from the remainder of the topics discussed in the book. What is it that gives you life? If you woke up tomorrow with unlimited money, what would you want to do with the rest of your life?

Imagine that the world has ended. One exercise to help you

determine what you find to be most important is to imagine the things that you would be perfectly fine living without. If you only had ten minutes to pack a bag that you'd be carrying with you forever, what do you decide to take?

Fact-Checking Your Feelings

A crucial step in this process of learning faster and more efficiently is understanding the difference between your response and your emotions. We all have emotions that we feel. They are natural and we can't always help them. The thing that you can help, however, is your response to these emotions. You are entirely in charge of the methods that you choose to respond to the feelings that you have throughout the day.

What gets in the way of clear thinking is often our unmanageable emotions. How many people can you think of who have seriously altered their life by acting impulsively on emotions? Maybe there's that person that quit their job after one bad day. Perhaps someone was feeling angry at their partner, so they cheated in the heat of the moment. There are split-second reactions that can have good outcomes, but if we're not careful, they can be way more destructive than productive in the end.

Anger blinds you. It makes it difficult to see the reality of the situation, and often you'll create your kind of perspective around a situation that might anger you. Rather than understanding what went on, it can be easy to place blame and only see things from one perspective.

Regret can keep you stuck in the past. Anxiety makes you worried over the future. Jealousy causes you to only look at the things you don't have. As you can see, some of these more challenging emotions can have serious effects on your overall ability to think cognitively and efficiently.

In order to think clearly, you have to understand the cognitive distortions that keep you from having an overall healthy mentality. Let's take a look at the kinds of thoughts, which are hindering your ability to think clearly, quickly, and critically.

One common cognitive distortion is the "all or nothing" mentality. This is the idea that because something can be labeled in one way, that means that it has every definition of that specific stereotype. For example, if you met someone that came from prison, you might assume they were a criminal. This is the "all or nothing" mentality, because, in your mind, they are a criminal, even if they are not.

This is similar to the "black-or-white" style of thinking. There is a whole gray area in between much of what we know that can explain a lot of the things that we might not understand initially. Black-or-white thinking means that if something is one way, that means that it can only be that way, and there's no in-between. If you woke up and the first thing you read was a terrible news story about a murder, then you could assume the world is a terrible place because of the tragedy. It is true that the instance is sad, but one moment doesn't define an entire world.

Personalization is also frequently toxic to thinkers that want to have the chance to understand the deep truth. This is when you put your own perspective into every situation. Did you walk by a group of people that were laughing? They must have been laughing at you, right? Did two of your friends hang out without you? They must be trying to cut you out of your life. These thoughts aren't true, but it is the way that we use personalization in our thinking. It is a pattern of thought that causes us to believe that everyone is out to get us and wishes to affect us directly.

Some individuals will always believe that they are right. Even when proven wrong, they can quickly come up with a reason as to why they were wrong or why they might have felt that particular way. Have you ever proven someone wrong and they said, "Well, I didn't know," or "You misunderstood me." This happens; however, it is also true that people are wrong a lot. There's nothing wrong with being wrong! However, many individuals believe admitting fault means that they are not intelligent. This plays into the all-or-nothing category as well. Some believe they have to be right all the time because that one moment of being wrong would disrupt all the other instances that they have shown intelligence.

Placing blame can clog your thinking. It means that you are giving power to other people and that they have control over how you might act or feel. Not every situation is one that warrants the need to place blame.

If you aren't checking in with your feelings, then it will make it harder to know what's going on in a situation. You won't be able to think clearly with cognitive distortions because you are altering perspective. You can't think critically if you don't think clearly, and you won't be able to think fast, either, if you don't stay in touch with your emotions and how you feel. Remember to keep track of your cognitive distortions to overcome any toxic thought patterns!

Common Mistakes of Clear Thinkers

Once you start to practice these methods, you will discover that you can already see a difference in the level of clarity when you start to think. It is never easy to admit that you are wrong, and not everyone realizes how negatively they might be forming perspectives. The sooner that you can recognize these mental faults, the easier it is to overcome them so that you can have the best brain possible! Let's take a look at a few more mistakes that you might run into along the path of becoming a more level-headed person and discover ways that you can get around these bigger issues.

One mistake is having a closed-off mind. This frequently occurs when we make assumptions and stick to stereotypes. You are creating assumptions based on things that you already know. That is fine and normal. What isn't healthy is making definitive statements. You see someone walking down the street and they have tattoos, piercings, black clothing, and a mean look on their face. Stereotypes have taught us that these types of people are tough, mean, and have other negative attributes. Maybe they are! Maybe they do have a tough exterior, and if you think of that as they are walking by you, that doesn't mean you are a bad person. However, a closed-off mind will use this knowledge and assume that they are a bad person. Someone with an open mind is aware of the stereotypes, but they would never let this instance be a defining moment for them. They wouldn't draw a conclusion about this person until they got the chance to talk to them and know them.

Clear thinking happens when we push past the illusions that have been created. These illusions might have been put in place by outside sources like the media, our parents, and society in general. If you learn how to push past these illusions, then you will be able to think more clearly. When you have a thought, ask yourself where it came from. Is this a conclusion that you drew on your own, or is it something that has been taught to you by outside sources?

It is natural for us to avoid threats, but we often do this to the point that we miss out on a positive opportunity that might be waiting. Just because something is risky, or it might scare you doesn't mean that you should avoid this. In fact, if it scares you, that means it could be something good for you in the end. We will talk more about these types of mental traps and how to avoid them when we discuss accelerated learning.

Throughout the rest of the book, we will be providing you

with more practical applications of clear thinking rather than focusing on the cognitive distortions that might already exist within you. It is up to you to make sure that you are checking in with your true feelings. Look deep within yourself and never be afraid to seek the truth.

[2]
HOW TO BE MORE PRODUCTIVE

Studies have shown that emotional regulation will play a factor in our desire to procrastinate (Pychyl, 2019). When you don't have a good handle on managing your emotional response, the chances of you struggling to find motivation and avoid procrastination are going to be higher as well. Sometimes it feels like we fall into the same patterns of thought over and over again. How many times have you woken up in the morning, exhausted, thinking to yourself, "Tonight I'm going to bed early." Then you get home, go to get ready for bed, and you end up staying up late all over again, only to repeat the same process the next day. The thing that gets in the way of our productivity the most is our brain.

The shape of our brain is different when we frequently procrastinate. This is why it can be challenging to have a productive mind. Not only do we think differently because of our motivational levels, but it plays a role in the way that our noggins have formed! This tells us that the more you procrastinate, the more likely you are to procrastinate even further. We have that motivation to not procrastinate. We have that desire to live a productive life. Actually, putting in the work towards that mindset is the difficult challenge that often keeps us from getting what we want.

There are certainly other factors that play into why we are able or not able to have an efficiently working mind. You are already aware of some unhealthy habits you might have that get in the way of procrastinating. Rather than discussing the "why" of procrastination, let's look at the "how" of the methods that will enable you to think more efficiently and accurately to increase your personal productivity.

Thinking More Efficiently and Accurately

We all know how to think, but not everyone is aware of how to think with efficiency and accuracy. Throughout your day, you have a ton of thoughts. They're pretty much endless. What those who don't think efficiently do is let their thoughts scare them. They will think of an idea and sometimes let that drive them throughout the next week. It can be easy to get an idea in your head one minute and let this become your life the next. Then there are individuals who will let their fantasies become the daydream that writes their life story. If you want to stop letting your thoughts take over and be the efficient and accurate thinker needed, it is time to turn this flow of thoughts around. There are some practical methods that you have to be aware of as well.

You have to understand how different things might make your brain less efficient. We have to be aware of the physical things we do for our health which might be clouding our judgment.

First, make sure that you are getting the right amount of sleep. Sleep is necessary because it is time for your brain to recharge. All throughout the day, your arms, legs, torso, and head are moving around. Your eyes look at things and process them. You take in new information constantly, even when you are sitting at home doing nothing. Sleep is your brain's chance to shut off so that it can come back even more refreshed tomorrow. If you are not giving your brain that right amount of sleep, it is not going to work, as simple as that. Some people will wonder why their mind works the way it does as they only get four to six hours of sleep a night. This also happens after sitting on their phone and staring at a bright screen for the minutes leading up to bed. Rather than doing this, make sure that you instead give yourself at least seven hours of distraction-free sleep a night. Go to bed on time. If you need seven hours of sleep and have to wake up at 7 a.m., then go to bed at 11:30 p.m. If you go to bed at midnight, you aren't giving yourself those full hours, and you will get more tired faster after already waking up with not having enough sleep.

Eating a healthy diet is also an essential step. The foods that we eat and the things we consume will directly affect the way our brain operates. We need important health foods to ensure that we are giving our brain proper vitamins and nutrients needed to function optimally.

Try to avoid excessive sugar or refined carbohydrates. These contain a ton of glucose, and too much can be hard for your body to process. Rather than using this sugar as energy, your body stores it, so even though your brain needs food, it might not be getting enough from your body if all you eat are these high in fat or sugary foods.

Understand the factors that can contribute to inflammation. Inflammation is your body's response to outside sources that could be damaging to your overall health. Think of the last time you got a cut or scrape on your skin. It likely swelled up and was red, maybe even itchy afterward. This is because your body is trying to fight off anything that might end up hurting it. This doesn't happen on your skin; it is happening inside your body as well. Too many additives and other inflammatory foods could cause your brain to become inflamed, making it harder for it to function.

Exercise is important for your body. It increases dopamine and serotonin, two things that are incredibly important for having a happy and healthy mind. If you aren't exercising, it is going to end up hurting your brain in the end.

Remember to keep all parts of health in check. Anything from diabetes to depression could affect the way that your mind works. Go to your doctor regularly, and if you really struggle with your cognition to an extreme level, it is time to talk to a professional to make sure there isn't any underlying issue that's making this difficult.

Social interaction is also important for your brain health. You have to talk to other people and talk out loud, in order to increase cognitive function. Talking to other people means that we are expressing our ideas. It also helps us to learn more as we discuss certain things with them. Think of how you might have thought something before, and then you said it out loud only to think, "That sounded better in my head." This is because social interaction helps to remind us of the boundaries that exist within our world and forces us to evaluate our thoughts.

You could have all the resources ever needed to have stronger thinking. However, if you don't pay attention to these pillars of brain health, you still won't be able to think entirely cognitively. We are creatures that have biological makeup that can't always be affected by the way that we think.

Use Negative Thoughts for Positive Results

Our most challenging thoughts can feel like the ones that are useless to us. What good does feeling angry or jealous all the time do? What has your constant misery done for you? While it can seem like these types of feelings are pointless, there is a lot within them that we can use to discover about ourselves. If you want to have more productive thinking, then rather than believing that you have to cut negative emotions out of your life, learn the ways that you will be able to use them for good. How can you take this kind of thought and turn it around so that it is more productive? What can be gained from having this kind of emotion?

The first thing that negative emotion is going to do is give you insight into a deeper thought or feeling that you have. It will let you know deeper things about yourself that you might not have realized in the first place. Our thoughts are like icebergs. While you can see a small top above water, there is a massive chunk of ice hidden beneath the surface that accounts for the majority of the mass of the iceberg.

There are certain things that we can only experience after going through a situation first. For example, you might never be able to appreciate your health until it is threatened. How many times have you been sick and thought to yourself how much you miss the ability to breathe through your nose? Was there ever a time when you broke a bone and struggled to use that body part? Though these challenging emotions can be hard, we can be productive with them by reminding ourselves of all that we have to be grateful for.

Let these emotions remind you that you are human. They are things that you can use to connect with other people. They give you a chance to reflect on your past and experiences to find a greater truth to yourself. You might only realize how important a period of time or a person was in your life after this instance has already occurred.

Some of the feelings will help us when it comes to assisting others. Maybe you are a parent with growing children. One day, they might get to a point where they can't think clearly, struggle with depression, or suffer from chronic anxiety. Not just our children, but friends and other family members can experience these things as well. If you've gone through them first, it will help you relate to them so that the two of you can end up helping each other.

Everything that we've been through has made us who we are today. Although some of it might have been an intense struggle, each moment of your life has played an important role in creating the person that you have become. All of the experiences you've had are things that directly impact your future. Though it hasn't been easy, we can still be grateful for the hard stuff because it has brought us some of the good we have in our lives now.

Use this method of negative emotion -> positive result whenever possible. It will help you think more critically and give you a chance to have a clear head on your shoulders.

Prioritize Your Thoughts

As we already mentioned, there are hundreds, possibly thousands, of thoughts that pass through your head on a daily basis. Some are good, some are bad. Sometimes these thoughts will become the thing that determines our next move. You might have a thought like, "I'm a disappointment and not doing anything with my life." This could have two results. It could inspire you to be better, or it could make you feel worse so that you participate in unhealthy habits once again. If you have a healthy thinking routine, then you can start to make sure that you use these challenging thoughts to be more productive. In order to have a healthy thinking routine, here is an exercise for you to try.

Start to prioritize your thoughts. What is most important for you to think about every single day? You can't be productive if you don't have your priorities straight. Which thoughts are the ones that are going to bring you to the things that you want most from this life? How are you going to be able to work through the things that cause you pain for better and more efficient results?

List your thoughts by what is most important. These should include positive thoughts. They should be creative and productive patterns that help inspire and motivate you throughout your day. Whenever you have a negative thought, you will know that it is not to be prioritized, so you won't spend as much time on it. Which thoughts bring you the most productivity?

The most productive thoughts are ones that are actionable plans of what you need to do next. The least productive ones are those that keep you in a different world. If you are thinking of fantasies of what your life is going to look like in ten years, this is a nonproductive thought. It is good to think of the future, but there's no need to play out entire scenes in your head.

The best thoughts are those which will help you to grow and learn even more. Focus on the moment now, and you will get those things you are fantasizing about in the end. You can never achieve your dreams if all your time is spent simply dreaming. These are the ones that should be at the top of your list. Use the same method for your tasks as well. Make a list of the most important at the top and the least important at the bottom, then start from the top down.

Try to have one large overall goal. What is it that you want from your life more than anything? What is one thing you would be disappointed to tell your childhood self that you never accomplished? If you were on your deathbed, what would be your last effort? After you come up with an overall goal, break it down. What needs to be done each year? What do you have to do every month? How is this going to affect what you do on a daily basis?

Make your schedule on a 24-hour basis, with a loose idea for the week. If you try to plan your week down to the very last second, it will be harder to follow through. If you create a schedule where you do one thing at 8:00, then one thing at 8:10, then another at 8:15, that's a great organization, but it is not going to set you up for success. What happens is you might miss that thing at 8:10, and the thing at 8:15 takes you more time than you thought. Then the rest of your day has been derailed, and you might end up feeling bad about yourself because you didn't accomplish what you thought. Have a list of ideas and prioritize what's most important rather than trying to plan too meticulously.

Remember to give yourself a break. Prioritize stress relief!

We often only think about creating schedules for the harder tasks, but you have to make sure to set time aside to relax. If we continue to forget about relaxing over and over again, we will never give ourselves the chance to have those cool-down periods.

[3]

FAST FOCUS AND BETTER CONCENTRATION

It is natural for your brain to want to wander off. Even when you are trying to pay attention actively, your brain will still wander around. Part of this is a survival skill. Think about how if you let a dog loose in a new home, it will run around and sniff as much as possible. It is gathering information. It is looking for clues and gaining a sense of its surroundings. This sort of discovery is natural and helps it to sniff out threats or even food. We have this sort of natural curiosity as well. Our brains crave something different when we sit for too long because it needs constant stimulation to function. However, if we let this curiosity get out of control, it can make it incredibly hard to focus and concentrate.

Building focus is essential, and there are many benefits that research has shown to help emphasize the importance of increasing this cognitive function (Hasenkamp, 2013). When you can increase your focus, it gives you a better chance of having a higher level of efficiency when completing a task. We often think that multitasking is cool and that you are smarter if you can do more than one thing at once. In reality, we end up splitting our attention and make it so that we are less concentrated on each thing that we do. Having more focus and a higher level of concentration will also help your memory, ensuring that you remember important information as you are learning about it.

The most important thing you can do is to bring your focus back to whatever it is that you have wandered away from. The benefits that we mentioned previously were from a study conducted by Hasenkamp that studied breathing in various participants. When they focused on their breathing, it helped keep their attention. Eventually, they would lose focus and wander off in their thoughts. To bring the focus back, they had to recognize first that they had wandered. The more focus that was put into staying concentrated on breathing, the less time was spent wandering. The mind drifting away still happened and always will. What's important is that we bring that focus back each time as quick as possible rather than letting those thoughts take us completely off-road. Think of your mind like a car going down the highway. You are going to drift a little bit left and a little bit right in between the painted lines, and you can never drive perfectly straight. This is natural, but you always know how to straighten your wheel and make sure that you keep moving forward, at the very least staying in between the lines. The dangerous part comes in when you drive completely off-road to the point that you can't even make it back to the main highway! Your thoughts will always wander like how you drift as you are driving. Put an emphasis on making sure you don't drive off-road, but don't expect to never drift at least a bit. Let's discuss some methods and tricks to make your concentration and focus much stronger.

Stop Multitasking

If you are reading this because you want to be more productive and think faster, you might be assuming that you need to learn how to do more than one thing at a time. Multitasking sounds like the best option for many who want to be more efficient and have the ability to accomplish as much as possible. However, it is the opposite.

Multitasking can be more damaging to your time. This is because you are taking all the concentration and focus that you have and end up splitting it between several different things. Imagine that you have ten kids and you need to teach them all an important lesson. You would think that teaching them all at once is the best way to do it. This is how many schools are set up. However, in the process, you lose the attention of one, another doesn't understand what you are talking about, two end up talking among each other, and the rest of the kids struggle to follow along. It takes you about ten minutes to teach the lesson, but then you have to spend twenty minutes with each re-explaining what was taught. It would be faster to spend that individual time with those students because while you are teaching one, the rest could discuss what the lesson was about and develop their ideas better! The thing about multitasking is that it's quantity over quality. That's not going to help you as you are learning! Instead, it is going to create surface-level information that's harder to retain.

Distraction can actually affect your IQ (Bregman, 2010)! If you aren't making sure to keep a clear mind, it will get in the way of your ability to better remember certain aspects of information. The best strategy to learn more clearly is to give as much of your attention to one thing as you can. Let's think of a real example of this. Say you are a pastry chef decorating cookies. You try to multitask by icing three different styles of cookies at once. What ends up happening when you multitask is that you spread your attention, so that each cookie then wouldn't be getting the right amount of care. It can cause sloppy work, and as you are moving through the different cookies, you are confusing your brain. You might end up mixing up icing or patterns because you are trying to remember how to complete each task.

Stop multitasking, no matter how much you want to. Split up your tasks by most important to least important, and then include how long each of them will take. You should strive to complete your most important tasks first, but if this is a challenge, then you can start instead by splitting them up by time. Here's an example of a to-do list for a Saturday, from most important to least important:

· Pay bills (15 minutes)

· Study (2 hours)

· Feed the dog (5 minutes)

· Workout (30 minutes)

· Respond to boss's email (5 minutes)

· Put laundry away (10 minutes)

As you can see, the most important thing to do for the day is to pay bills and study. If you don't pay your bills, bad things happen like late fees and getting the internet or electric cut off! Animals are our responsibility, so we have to remember to feed them. Working out is important for your health and skipping that could mean skipping it the next day and the next day and so on. Obviously, you need to respond to your boss and put laundry away, but if you don't get these things done, you could do them Sunday.

However, some people might look at this list and feel over-whelmed. They might not feel like studying, so that gets pushed back, meaning all other tasks get pushed back. To think more efficiently and increase productivity, you could try to reprioritize your list. Maybe you do it by things that will take the least amount of time rather than the most important. Then this would be the order of your list:

· Feed the dog

· Respond to boss's email

· Put laundry away

· Pay bills

· Workout

· Study

If you did this, you would be able to knock out over half your list within the time it would have taken you to complete the first few things on your initial list. This is important for your brain because, after 30 or so minutes, there would be two things on your to-do list left rather than the initial five there would have been if you did things in order of importance. While you still have the same things to do for the day, it can help your brain be more prioritized if you focus on knocking out small tasks to boost your confidence and make you feel good about yourself.

Give yourself shorter deadlines. When you stop multitasking, it means that you can get one thing done faster. Give yourself extremely short deadlines for each individual task so that you feel more pressure to focus your attention and get it all done within that restricted time period.

Multitasking can still help if it is going to be beneficial for the projects not for your time frame. If multitasking means that you are able to knock out two things at once because they're similar but require different parts of your brain, then go for it. For example, if you have to listen to a speech for a class and fold your laundry, these are things that you could do at the same time. The laundry is easy because it's physical. You have to fold clothes. The speech is more mental. What you wouldn't want to multitask is listening to the speech while trying to write a report for another project, as these things are both mental.

Get Rid of Mental Distractions

Your mind is going to be a bit distracted, even when you are doing your best! Whether it's the thoughts of what made you anxious earlier that day, a fear that you have over the future, or something else that is causing you agony, it's important to check in with your mental distractions to determine what you can do better to give you a clearer mind.

First, remember that you should clear up physical distractions. If you have a garage with half-finished projects, crafts sitting around uncompleted, dishes that need to be done, a messy floor covered in cat hair, and so on, then you will want to make sure that you clean these up if you are going to be focusing on something in that space. Even though you might be able to push these things out of your mind momentarily so that you don't think about them, your eyes still see them. Each time you look at something, your brain still takes a bit of energy to process that bit of information.

Keep your space clutter-free to give your brain a better chance at having the same level of mentally clarity.

Work through your emotions and understand how to manage them. Even though you might be far away from your family that caused stress over the weekend, that doesn't mean that your mind is free from emotions. You have to clean up your mental space as much as you clean up your physical space for optimum cognition.

Let patience be your main focus. If you can't stay patient and in the moment, then that is because there are thoughts distracting you. Are you anxious that something isn't happening fast enough? Are you worried about the outcome? Are you fearful that something bad is going to happen? Are you angry that you aren't getting enough attention? Are you frustrated that you are not doing something else? The strategy to fight through patience is to make sure that you are aware of what it is that is making you so aggravated with the present moment.

Know the difference between things that you can control, influence, and have no power over at all. If you want to increase your focus, you have to know how to concentrate on the things that you can influence. Far too often people think that they can change certain things which they have no control over at all! If you focus all your time and energy on fixing something unfixable, then you are wasting precious moments that could be concentrated on other things.

Don't ruminate over the past. Keep your thoughts productive. It's good to be reflective, but you shouldn't be sitting there thinking, "I wish I had done this, I should have done that, I could have changed that," and so on. Instead, you can think, "In the future, I'll do this, I know now not to do that, I have the ability to affect my future by doing this." You don't want to shut the past out, but since it can't be changed, there's no point wishing that we could.

One strategy you can use is to give yourself mental time to reflect. Try to notice what you did throughout a day. Maybe you journal it, or you can share it with someone else. Whatever works best for you is fine, just put attention on going through your day mentally to see your strengths, weaknesses, the good, and the bad.

Remember to check in with your cognitive distortions consistently. If you really want to improve your brainpower and take your mind to unexpected places, it is essential that you start to find methods of cleaning up your brain.

Concentration Exercises

The biggest distraction of all might simply be that you are too stressed to understand what you have to get done. There are things in the way of you having complete and total concentration. Some of the mental habits that you have might be the direct thing that is making it so hard to focus. If you don't know what your problem with focus is, you won't know how to improve on it.

To have better concentration, we have a few exercises that

you can try to do. These are things that you can do anytime, anywhere, to give you an idea of the mental hurdles you will have to jump over to have improved focus.

One method is to do a "wall sit." This is when you place your back flat against a wall and use your legs to hold you up as if you were sitting on a chair. It's very challenging and can cause strain within your legs. It is a physical exercise that many do for health, but it can help you with your mental health as much. When you are wall sitting, you will be confronted with the things that make it hard for you to focus. Are you thinking of the pain? Are you worried about falling? Are you stressed because you are uncomfortable? While you are doing this, simply ask yourself these questions. Look deep within yourself to discover what it is that's making this particular exercise so challenging. Why can't you simply sit against the wall for a long period of time? You will discover your biggest concentration weaknesses within this exercise.

For a second concentration exercise, we're going to focus on your eye's ability to pick up on different objects that are in plain view. Have three different objects in three different places. This would mean having something right in front of you, something about five feet or so away, and something farthest from you across the room. Take thirty seconds with each item to stare at it and focus on it as if your eyes were a camera lens. Take a minute to study this object, and then switch your focus to the one behind it. After you make it to the item that's farthest away, bring your attention back to what was right in front of it. This gives you the chance to see your eye's ability to focus on different objects. While you are physically focusing, you are also increasing your brain's ability to focus mentally. You can study the object and try to pick up on as many details as possible, ignoring the other two objects that are also in that field of vision.

Make eye contact with yourself when talking in a mirror. When we talk in front of the mirror or are practicing a speech, it's easy to look at all other parts of our body. Maybe we stare at our hair, our outfit, our body, and our hands. Next time you have a presentation or speech, practice in front of the mirror and only look into your eyes. You will be amazed at how much this increases concentration and focus.

Hold your breath for 10-15 seconds while doing something simple. This is something like doing the dishes, chopping vegetables, switching laundry, washing your hair, and so on. Nothing that could be dangerous if you had your breath held. Take a big breath in as you count for 10, hold your breath for 10 seconds (or as long as you can if you can't make it to 10), and then breathe out for 10. You will notice that while you hold your breath, you are able to turbo-focus on what you are doing! This isn't an activity to replace the methods that you use to do other things, because holding your breath for prolonged periods is dangerous. It's just a quick and simple way to help you bring the concentration back in the moment and become aware of how much you might have not been paying attention.

Make sure that you check in with your posture and your desire to fidget or move around a ton. If your leg is shaking uncontrollably, stop it, walk around for a minute, and sit back down. If you are slouching, make sure to sit up straight. Eventually, you'll likely slouch again, but it's important to keep checking in with our physical focus so that we can mentally concentrate easier.

[PART 2]
THINK CRITICAL

[4]
WHAT IS CRITICAL THINKING?

Everyone on this planet can benefit from improving their critical thinking skills. Critical thinking sounds serious. When you say that someone is in critical condition, you often associate them with being in the intensive care unit or having other serious health conditions. When we are talking about critical thinking, this is in reference to the way in which we are able to analyze a situation, thought, or other subjects to the best of our ability in order to create a perception or judgment around this studied area. If someone asked you "How many people live in your city?" you could Google the answer. If you were going to think about this critically, you might consider how many houses are on your street, the average size of the household, how many people might be in an area per block, and so on. You would look at every last detail and analyze this material in order to come up with your comprehensive answer.

If you are not a critical thinker, you put yourself at risk for becoming more manipulated by others easily. Those who lack critical thinking skills are the ones that "go with the flow." They will take things at face value and accept the new information presented to them for what it is, not making any personal judgments of their own. This isn't bad in all situations. Not everything has to be overthought. However, it is dangerous when you don't critically think about new and important information presented to you. Think of those who only base their news off headlines from one news source. At the top of many news articles, there are bulleted lists about what the source contains. This is helpful for quick thinking, but many individuals only use this as their main source of information. A critical thinker knows how to read through the whole article, cross-check the information with other sources, and to look at the actual references and citations used in order to draw their conclusion.

Critical thinking is the way that we can discover a greater truth. It is how we are able to question someone else's beliefs. It is when we can say, "Are you sure about that?" or "Where are you getting that information?" to make others question their knowledge. It is how great conversations are formed and incredible discoveries are made.

You are in charge when you are thinking critically. When you wake up, brush your teeth, go to the bathroom, hop in the shower, and get your morning coffee, none of this requires critical thinking. When you are at work, problem-solving and coming up with new solutions, this is when you want to put more of an emphasis on critical thinking. If you want to think critically about those menial tasks, more power to you! Everything can be investigated for greater truth and deeper meaning, so let's take a look at the methods that you can do this now!

How to Understand Thought Biases

To think critically, you first want to identify the restrictions of your thoughts that already exist. There are certain biases that we have which will guide the things that we think. These biases have been created first by the people that raised you. Whether it was a grandparent, aunt or uncle, sibling, or your parents, the people that shared ideas with us as we grew up will certainly have a large role in the things that we think now.

Remember the things that you were taught to not only believe but emphasize as you were a child. Some of our parents value money. Some value looks. It wasn't that they necessarily taught you this directly, but you might have picked up on this throughout your life. For example, think of two girls from the same neighborhood, one with a single mother and one with two parents that have a little more money. That girl from a single mother might place more of an emphasis on having and making money than the other girl because that was her mom's main focus. Financial struggles were a part of the stress of the family for the single mother and her daughter, so the girl learned that this is an important part of life that needs to be focused on. The girl from the married parents with good jobs never had to worry about money a day in her life, so she won't focus on this as she gets older.

Stop considering that you were able to "predict" what happened. After something happened, we often think to ourselves, "I knew that was going to happen." This is true, but because you probably predicted both outcomes. For example, imagine that you invited a friend to your party. This friend frequently flakes out and doesn't come even though they sometimes say they will be there. In your mind, you are assuming they are going to skip the party, but a part of you knows that they might still come. Let's say that they do come to the party. You might say, "I knew this time would be the time that they came!" But then in a different situation, they don't show up. You might then say, "I knew that this was going to happen." Before a situation occurs, you likely have multiple ideas of what will happen. Then when a situation occurs, you will have "predicted" it because you knew that there were only so many options for what could happen. If you had to pick an outcome and stick with that one situation, we would often "predict" a lot less.

The first thing that you hear might sometimes be the thing that you believe. If someone walks into a room and the first thing that you think is, "What are they wearing? They look ridiculous." That doesn't mean that is how you feel. This might have been the way that you were taught to think by a family memory or other authority figure. It is usually the thought that comes after that shows your true character.

We often jump to conclusions. Rather than doing this, it is important that we instead make a note of improving our ability to inference. One study showed that we are more likely to think we predicted something than to predict it (Cherry, 2019). This study looked at individuals who predicted the outcome of an election. Before, around 50% voted that one candidate would win. Then the candidate won, and they were asked if they had predicted this would happen. More than 70% said they predicted it, even though less than that had initially. This shows us that we use assumptions and predictions too frequently.

We look for things to validate the perspective that we already have. There are certain beliefs and values that you already know to be true. If you aren't aware of these things, it means that you will end up hurting yourself in the end because you aren't thinking outside of certain thought biases. To think critically, make yourself aware of the boundaries that restrict you to give yourself a better chance of freeing up your thoughts.

Remember that sometimes, we mix up our thoughts and memories. Your memory is going to be based on your perspective. Just because you thought a situation was scary, or even fun, that doesn't mean that's how everyone felt at the time. Though you can reflect and use your memory for more important information, there are still moments where you have to check in with yourself and ask, "Did that really happen how I thought it did?"

Know that you have a predisposed idea of a person the moment that you meet them. It's not our fault, but we often will judge someone based on how they look right away. It is a way that we were taught. Messy hair and a stain on a shirt might mean they are sloppier. Expensive shoes mean that they have money. A smile means they're friendly. A squeezed brow means that they're angry. These things could be true, but we can't associate these things with visual cues every time because there are so many instances where it's not true at all.

Not everyone is going to be able to understand and comprehend what you mean in your words either. No matter how much you might try to explain yourself, we have to remember that others have just as many boundaries and restrictions on their thinking as we do. These are all important things to remember when we start to increase our ability to think critically.

Methods for Developing Critical Thinking

Critical thinking doesn't happen overnight. There are some steps involved to get you to a stage of critical thinking. You have been thinking a certain way for a large portion of your life already. Even though you might try rather hard, you won't be able to think differently tomorrow. There are patterns and habits that we are going to help you break through, but first, let's look at some actual methods to bring you into a clearer headspace. When you have the ability to think clearly, it gives you the chance to think critically. We discussed the ways you can free up mental space, so now let's do something with that free area!

First, you have to become aware of the way that you are failing to think critically now. What are those thought biases that we discussed? The basic attributes you have will create those boundaries. Your race, education, financial status, gender, sex, parental figures, religion, and so on are all things that create these boundaries of thought. Of course, two people who have different races, educations, financial statuses, and so on don't necessarily think differently. These are things that might alter your thought patterns.

Then there will be a stage of initial improvement. Once you have become aware of your critical thinking challenges, next you have the ability to start to improve on this in different ways. This is key to helping you think and grow better.

You might think that you have become a critical thinker, but then you start to understand all the things that you don't know. Truly, the more you know, the more you realize you don't know. Imagine that you found a new animal. This is unlike any other creature and it is a great discovery. The first thing you learned was that there is another animal. After that, these are all the things you have yet to learn:

1. What does it eat?

2.How often does it eat?

3.How does it get its food?

4.How many are there?

5.Where does it sleep?

6.How often does it sleep?

Knowing that there's a new animal means that you have more knowledge than others who have yet to make the discovery. However, once you unlock this new door of information, your journey isn't over! This is where critical thinking comes in. You become aware of knowledge, but then it becomes time to dig deeper! The first man on the moon didn't look at the moon and say, "Found it! We're done now!" That was the beginning of a long journey of learning.

Reflecting is going to be the most important thing you can do as a critical thinker. You probably want to learn fast, but you can't rush every new bit of information that you want to learn. One method to get you started is to make sure that you understand how you've made the most of the time that you have already. Look back on time in your life where you made a mistake. Maybe it's something you wish you hadn't done, or you feel like you've wasted time. Time is real! It can never be wasted! What happened in this time that made you the person you are now? How have you been able to learn from this?

Recognize one positive and one negative part of your day every day. Whether you are discussing this with the family during dinner, or you are lying in bed thinking about it, what is one good thing that you experienced, and what is something bad that you didn't enjoy? This is going to give you the best chance of critically thinking about your life.

Critical Thinking Strategies

Throughout the remainder of your time on this earth as a critical thinker, there are certain strategies that you will always want to attempt to include in your daily life. These are daily practices like brushing your teeth, taking a shower, and so on, that you should do naturally. The better you equip yourself to develop critical thinking strategies, the easier it is to learn faster, think clearer, and analyze more critically. These are seven strategies to learning and analyzing all new information that you take in.

Adapt to the situation. We have to remember the way that we might avoid certain situations because they are different. Whether you walked into your office to find you have a new manager, or you discovered that a belief you had turned out to be a lie, adapt. Don't try to change the situation. You can influence it eventually, but make sure that you are aware of how to adapt and accept things as they come to you first.

Strive for further truth. Dig deeper into the things that make you the most curious about. Refuse to accept anything at face value. Even if you did discover that it was the truth, after all, you might have picked up other important information.

Reflect on what you already know to be true. Just because you have had the same thought for 10 years doesn't mean that it is true. Go back and ask yourself where the root of your belief lies. Discover the potential for your brain and what might happen if you are able to combat these thoughts.

Inquire deeper into all that is presented to you. Like we mentioned with the discovery of a new animal, ask those follow-up questions to get a better understanding. Once you start exploring a new area, you might discover that there is nothing to support it, making it easier to know what info is important and what can be forgotten.

Create and create again. The first time you do something, it will not be the perfect way you can do it. The first time you do something, you might be better than others, but the second time you do something, you will be even better than yourself. The more that you focus on creating--whether you are creating a better life for yourself or simply painting a picture--the better you become in the end.

Talk about what you are learning. Don't hold it all in! When you discuss what you are learning with other people, you discover more truth about that subject, and you can validate or alter your beliefs around the subject.

Connect information in places that are seemingly opposites. Look for the individual strings that hold them together. Unleash the invisible associations that you can create. When you connect information, it makes it easier to understand.

As you start to make more connections, you unlock greater truth, you would never have discovered initially.

Not many people know how to think critically, nor will they throughout their lives. When these can become your mantras, your rules, and your objectives in life, you will better enable yourself to have that powerful mind you desire most.

[5]
HOW TO MAKE BETTER CHOICES

Every aspect of your life is one in which a singular choice could cause a ripple effect. Whether you make a decision surrounding your personal life or one that deals with a professional side, you'll have to make some tough choices throughout time. Having to make a decision can be one of the scariest things in life, but it is an essential part of our day-to-day living.

We all work for different things that we want for our future, and we have to find methods of strategizing in order to get these types of things. It isn't easy, which is why so many people are struggling. We often think that we couldn't help where we got in life. Sometimes we blame others, outside sources, and general fate for how we have ended up. However, our situation in life is mostly based on small individual choices that can affect the flow of how things unfold.

Your choices are influenced by your basic needs, as exemplified in Maslow's Hierarchy of Needs (Maslow, 1943). This evaluation proposes five levels of basic needs that we have, which have to be fulfilled. His theory proposes that you behave in a certain way based upon your needs. This hierarchy is presented in a pyramid.

At the very bottom are your basic physiological needs. These are things like food, water, and shelter or clothing. The shelter and clothing are necessary because we have a certain level of warmth that we need to survive. The food and water are also things that if we didn't have, we would literally die.

Next, you need safety and security. These are things like a home with locked doors, a bed we can count on every night, police to call when we are threatened, and other forces that help to make sure we feel protected.

Above this is the need for relationships, to belong and form bonds. These help you get the things that you want, which you cannot provide for yourself. Relationships help bring you to greater truths and give you the chance to learn more about yourself.

Second to the top are your esteem needs. This is the fulfillment that demands a sense of accomplishment. We all have to feel proud of ourselves and like we have done something. This gives you the chance to feel good with your own character, making life more fulfilling and bringing you to a greater truth.

At the very top is self-actualization. This is when you realize your potential and are able to fulfill this capability. Everything that you desire within this life can supposedly fall into one of these five categories.

Every choice that you make will then revolve around fulfilling one of these basic needs. If you want to start making better choices, then consider this hierarchy of needs to determine what it is that you are trying to fulfill. If your decisions have led you to a place where you don't think any of these are being met, then it is time to reevaluate your choices to improve your life. Let's look at a few other methods and strategies to help you make better choices.

How to Combine Logic and Creativity

There are two sides to your brain. One thinks logically, and one thinks more creatively. The logical side will analyze things, and the creative side will pay more attention to coming up with new ideas. Combining both of these gives you a better chance of increasing your motivation. We have to learn how to combine both logic and creativity if we want to make better choices. It can be hard to know how to choose the right things in life, but when we give everything a proper analysis using these methods, it will be easier to know what the best option can be.

Visualization is an important step in combining logic and creativity. This causes you to look ahead. Don't think of things that you hope will happen. Pay close attention to what can happen. What is likely to be the outcome based on things that you already know to be true? What past experience can help you determine the reality of a situation?

Next, determine which side of your brain it is that you are using more frequently. Are you more of a logical person? Do you think of reality, question people's choices and motivations, and dig for deeper truth? Are you more interested in discussing big ideas, new ways of doing things, and interesting innovations? When you can discover which side of your brain you are thinking with, it becomes easier to know what you need to improve on.

You have to start to build your intuition throughout life so that you can better judge a situation as it is presented to you. This intuition is something that we create as we continue to take in information. Intuition means that you know all possible outcomes and that you are accepting of anything that might come your way.

When we think of logic, math, science, and other factually based things, we often forget to be creative in the process. All of these areas crave creativity! How many boring math classes did you have to sit through? But how often do you use math elements now? It happens more frequently than you would have thought sitting in those classes, and life would be a bit simpler if we could easily come up with a percentage in our head, evaluate the loss/profit of a venture, or figure out what the tax on our grocery bill is going to be. Though this might have seemed like such a static subject, you can see through a real application of this information that a little creativity certainly would have helped to make it more interesting in the end.

Don't be afraid of a challenge that's presented to you. If you can't find a solution, then thinking creatively is what you need. When you start to think one way or the other, use the opposite side of your brain for a moment. If you have to come up with a new idea and you notice that you are only thinking of all the creative aspects, ground yourself by exploring the logical parts that need your attention the most. If you are only thinking logically and you can't seem to find a solution, consider the creative aspects that you are looking past.

When trying to make choices, we often stick to one way of thinking. If you have a creative issue, you assume it needs a creative solution. Don't limit yourself with these boundaries. Connect both sides of your brain for optimal results. Widen your knowledge and look at things that aren't so strictly associated with one side or the other.

Discover the beauty of nature. There is so much creativity and logic that occur naturally! Look at the way a tree grows. Logically it grows towards the sun, away from the ground. It develops a large trunk first, and then all the branches, and then the leaves. This is logical. Creatively, we can see how it grows to have these beautiful leaves. It casts gorgeous shadows onto the grass to create weird patterns. Look at all the ways that nature is presenting us with logic and creativity at the same time!

Always give yourself a brainstorming period for new ideas. Sometimes you might feel rushed and needed a solution fast, but even if it's ten minutes, give yourself some time. Go for a walk, take a shower, have a cup of coffee while you listen to some music. Do something to give yourself separation from the situation and the solution that you need to come up with.

All creative aspects and all logical aspects do incorporate each other. Nothing is 100% creative or 100% logical. There is certainly a weighted side to everything, but you can discover greater truth when you realize how both can work together.

Avoiding Manipulation Tactics

Sometimes, the reason that we struggle to make better choices is that we aren't aware of the way that we might be being persuaded one way or another over this decision. If you are in a group setting and you need to make better choices, you might discover that some people are the ones that have been influencing you. Not everyone has malicious intent with persuasion, but many individuals look out for their best interests first, so you might get forgotten along the way.

If you want to make better choices, you have to start by making sure that you are the one in charge. You should be the person that is able to decide the fate of your future. You shouldn't have to leave it up to someone else! Take control over your future and stop letting other people determine how you might think or act.

Researchers have studied methods of avoiding manipulation, and there are a few important lessons we can take away from these studies (Fransen, Smit, & Verlegh, 2015). You already resist some persuasion, but it's important to become aware of the methods by which you might be falling right into the hands of someone else.

There are usually two methods to avoid manipulation when influence is first detected. The first is to avoid persuasion. This might mean clicking on a news article that talks about the economy, only to stop reading after you discover there are certain biases in the writing.

The second method is to contest it. This would be to argue about the persuasion. Rather than clicking away, you might want to read the whole article then decide to comment or even contact the writer to argue about the things that were discussed.

If you don't even know you are being manipulated, how are you supposed to come up with a strategy? Of course, when we are feeling persuasion, it's easier to stop it as it's happening. It's the sneakier stuff that can make us feel as though our thoughts aren't our own. Again, not everyone knows that they're being persuasive, and they don't always have malice in their heart. However, they can still sway us, so we have to question their tactics to avoid manipulation.

Start by questioning the intention of the persuasion. Why is it that they might be wanting you to act in a certain way? If you can easily say, "So they don't have to do the work" or "So they can get what they want," it's obvious to see that they're trying to persuade you. If their intentions are for good and they are going to help both of you, then this is a sign that they are trying to do what's best.

Others might use certain manipulation tactics, like painting the situation in one way so that you don't see the negatives. They might invite you to their home turf so that you feel more inclined to agree to what they're proposing. They could end up using other persuasion tools, such as scarcity, to make you feel as though you need to jump on their offer before it's too late.

Understand the biases that many have which they will use to validate their perspectives. Social validation is another method of helping to bolster their attitude. Others might use the example that people agree with them to make their point seem more valid. For example, maybe someone is trying to get you to invest your money into a project. They might say, "Well, I've already gotten several offers from a few different people," as a way to make you feel as though socially, this is the right thing to do.

Check and ensure that your freedom isn't being threatened. If someone is trying to take away one of your basic human rights, then they might be trying to manipulate you. These are things like:

- the right to feel however you do
- the right to develop your own opinion
- the right to make your choices
- the right to object when you feel uncomfortable
- the right to think whatever you want

These are all things that no one should be allowed to take away from you. Empower yourself to stand up and always give yourself a chance to at least state your side. Demand that your opinion is validated among others.

Following Through and Sticking to Your Choice

The hardest part about making some choices is that we don't want to stick to them in the end! Even if it is something as simple as picking what you are going to watch on TV that night. There are some reasons behind why you might be so unsure of yourself even after you've managed to make a decision. The first one is because you lack the confidence to know that your thoughts and feelings are valid. You struggle to believe in your ability to make an intelligent and informed decision.

Confidence is key in making decisions. After you've given yourself the chance to come up with a solution and say "yes" to the answer you've created, then it will be up to you to make sure that you follow through with this decision. Don't back out because you are scared of what will happen. There are some strategies to help you follow through with whatever it is that you are deciding.

First, identify what might have happened that made it so difficult for you to make decisions and to be assured in yourself and your ability to make certain choices. If you grew up in a household where you never had a say in anything and others were always making decisions for you, this is going to play into your ability to feel confident now. If someone always made you feel silly about the decisions that you made, then this is also going to damage the way that you view your intelligence.

Sometimes you might feel frozen, unable to decide which option is best. This can be a fight or flight reaction. Rather than facing the thing that scares you (the decision), your brain decides to flee in order to avoid any mental strain or struggle that you feel in the process.

You have to start to trust yourself. You are the only person that you can 100% depend on for your entire life. Even if you trust someone entirely, they might not be there when you are picking out dinner at the store, choosing which college to go to, or helping you decide how to raise your children. Though others are trustworthy, you still have to trust yourself above all.

One method to help you improve your ability to make decisions is to use positive affirmations. Remind yourself throughout the day, "I can do this." We often say negative affirmations to ourselves like, "I'm not good enough," "Something always has to go wrong," or "Nothing will ever go my way." Instead, replace these with positive affirmations, such as:

· I am capable of anything.

· I have the ability to do this.

· Nothing is going to stop me from getting what I deserve.

· I am smart enough to know what's good for me.

· I am intelligent.

Destroy the belief that you are not good enough, smart enough, and so on. These aren't going to help you improve. Even if you have made terrible decisions and need to do a complete 180-degree change with the direction of your life, positivity is going to do so much better than the negativity that you might be experiencing.

Let others help give you advice, but don't put the decision making on anyone else. When you let others make important decisions for you, you are giving them power and control over your life. Only YOU are in charge of YOU.

Forgive yourself for decisions that you made in the past that you might not be as proud of now. The decisions that you made in the past do not have to affect the decisions you make about the future.

Remember that nothing terrible is going to happen if you make the wrong decision. Don't take everything so seriously.

Someone might be better, they might have had a different

solution, and maybe they would have overcome a problem that you had better. Stop thinking this way! Even if you do make a wrong decision, you will be able to learn something from this mistake, giving you a better chance to improve next time around. You can never improve if you never try in the first place!

The worst decision that you can make is to make no decision at all.

[6]

HOW TO STOP MAKING MISTAKES AND AVOID TRAPS

We think within a restricted boundary that keeps us trapped in the same toxic cycles over and over again. We're presented by the world, and from ourselves, the illusion of choice. What we don't realize is that we're often restricted by the same boundaries that we are trying to break free from. Critical thinking is the best way to pull you from these challenges to enable yourself to think more clearly and logically.

This chapter is going to provide you with logical and practical methods for overcoming your biggest mental tricks. These traps are patterns of thought that keep you from making the same mistakes over and over again. Sometimes you might question, "Why am I like this?" or "Why does this keep happening?" with no clear answer. There is a lot within your mind that can give you those clues; we have to know how to unlock them.

When you don't have a handle on your emotions, it can be like walking around a dangerous attic with creaky boards and loose holes. If you are not careful, you can fall right through the ceiling! It is essential we know how to overcome these mental traps. You have to be aware of your thoughts, the mistakes you've played a role in, and the mental traps you've fallen into in order to think more critically.

When you are raised to think a certain way, it will become your pattern of thought. Studies have proven that stressful life events will alter the way that you respond to stress in the future (Michl, Mclaughlin, Shepherd, & Nolen-Hoeksema, 2013). We've already discussed how you can start to separate your emotions from your reactions, but now it is time to apply that to heightened thinking. Not only can you manage your emotions, but you can use them to learn more about yourself. By doing this, you are giving yourself the best possible chance to think clearly and concisely.

We get used to certain thinking patterns. Sometimes, it is more comfortable to continue to think negatively or in a destructive way rather than trying to change our thought process. We become so used to the mental anguish we feel that we often forget that we are in charge of changing that. When you are spinning fast within a cycle, it is hard to pull yourself out and end these patterns.

Let's look at methods and strategies now to help remove you

from the mental traps that have you making the same mistakes over and over again.

How to Recognize Mental Cycles

If you are constantly making mistakes, especially the same mistakes, it is time to identify the mental traps that restrict you. There are many patterns of thought that we might possess, which can end up hindering our ability to think clearly and efficiently. Rather than letting yourself continually get caught up in the same mental traps, it's time to become fully aware of the cycles that you are spinning in.

It starts by recognizing the traps that are already there. Is it a family member that put these thoughts into your head? Was there someone in your life that always made it challenging for you to decide what was best for you?

You can't do the same thing that you have been doing and expect to get any different results from this process. If you want to change and grow, you have to come up with new methods to do so. If you grow a flower in a small pot, it is going to stay that same size until you give it a bigger pot to grow in. You can't expect something to change in the same place where the bad habits that require altercations live.

Absolutes are the fastest way to make you restrict the way that you are thinking. This is any kind of definitive statements, such as "I should do this," "I can't do that," "I'm always like this," "I'm never like that," and so on. These absolute phrases encompass several different factors but make one defining conclusion. If you are late for work three times in a month, then that is 17 out of 20 times that you were on time. However, that fourth time you are late, you might think, "I'm always running late." You can't use one moment to define all the moments.

Oftentimes, we start to create expectations over what might end up happening. We expect things to go as we planned out in our heads. We expect people to act in a certain way. This is a mental cycle that can consistently set you up for disappointment.

Comparisons can be mental traps that keep us from thinking critically. If you are always comparing yourself to other people, comparing progress, and so on, then it will make you feel inadequate. If you were to go online right now, you could probably find a picture of someone smiling because of success. Maybe they posted a picture with a new baby, or perhaps it's a friend who posts their graduation from college. They look happy, and at that moment when you view the picture, you might not be. Maybe you are sitting behind your desk at work or lounging on the couch. This comparison will make you feel inadequate. How could you compare a college graduate to someone binging a Netflix show they've already seen? You are not comparing in the right circumstance. That person who showed that picture is also showing the peak of their moments. They aren't going to post a picture of them having a mental breakdown in the bathroom because they studied for 12 hours straight. That person smiling with their baby won't post a picture of them struggling to go to the bathroom after giving birth. The comparisons we make are unfair to ourselves, so we have to recognize this mental cycle.

Have more productive conversations, not competitive ones. There are too many individuals that have discussions in which they turn the conversation into a competition. It's healthy to debate, and arguing over certain topics can help you to learn more. However, conversations should never be about "winning." A convo where one person is right and the other is wrong isn't going to do anyone any good. A conversation where both parties share their feelings, get insight into their thoughts, and positively persuade each other is one where both parties can "win."

Sometimes, we think that other people might be out to get us. It's easy to believe that everyone cares about themselves more than us and that others only want to hurt us. Although this is another mental trap because it is not the truth. Most people will put themselves first, but that is a survival instinct. If we assume that others don't care about us because they aren't putting our interests first, then that is a fault in our ego. If you make the realization that you are responsible for yourself and no one else is, then you will start to limit the thinking that others only wish to harm you.

A big mental trap that many individuals find themselves in is one where they focus more energy on pleasing other people than they do taking care of themselves. It's good to be an accommodating person, and we should strive to help others.

However, if you are taking care of other people's needs more frequently than you are checking in with your own, you are going to exhaust your brainpower in the end.

Don't make yourself feel guilty over the things you couldn't accomplish. Notice if there is a situation that triggers a certain response. To overcome these mental traps, you have to be aware of the deeply ingrained thoughts which are driving these intentions.

Unlock the secrets that you have been keeping from yourself. Have you been lying to yourself about a greater truth that needs uncovering? Maybe you are trapped in a loveless marriage, but you've convinced yourself it's not that bad because dealing with the mediocrity is easier than the fear of leaving. Perhaps you are already on track down a certain career path that you realized you hate, but you stick to it because it's easier than starting over again. Don't let your-self stay trapped inside your mentality!

Don't be afraid of change. Sometimes, change is terrifying. It can paralyze us. This is because we have to start to learn all over again. We have to evaluate new information and draw conclusions from this. We have to prepare for the unexpected and hope that everything goes as planned. Accept that this is going to be challenging at times. You are a work in progress after all! Be open to change, open to learning, and excited for new experiences. The more you practice this, the easier it will be to break the chains of your mind that have been restricting your thoughts.

Expectations and Goals

A big mental trap we make is having goals that are way too high. It's so easy to set goals. You literally just have to think of what you want and say that you are going to do it by a certain time. The problem is that many people set unattainable goals! When you start to set unrealistic goals, then you aren't going to get the things that you have been desiring the most.

We often create expectations that are unrealistic as well. We assume that everything is going to go perfectly. We expect people to act in a certain way. We hope that people know what we want and that they'll be able to give that to us.

To start, remember that nothing is ever going to turn out like you think it will. Even if you planned everything perfectly down to the last detail, there are going to be some things that get in the way and make this end up not happening. There will always be a level of uncertainty. Even if things do go exactly as planned, you are going to feel different throughout the process. We can never predict the way that we are going to feel on any given day because there are so many biological, internal, and external factors that will play into this.

Let the excitement be fun, but don't let it be the only fun part. Think of going on a vacation. Half the fun is the journey there, preparing, and becoming excited about the trip. If you build it up too much, however, you will be disappointed in the end. Remember that planning is fun, but don't let it be the only time that you experience joy throughout the process.

When we have goals and expectations that are too high, all it does to us is make us feel as though we're failures. If you create an impossible goal, then you won't make it, and you will feel bad about yourself. We end up wishing for perfection and when we can't get it, we blame ourselves. It's easy to say, "I want to lose 30 pounds this month." Anyone could say that. That's a completely unrealistic expectation, as it would mean losing a pound a day!

Recognize the ways that you might be putting expectations on other people. Maybe you have a struggle in a romantic relationship, and you hope that the other person notices this and that they'll change accordingly. You can't expect them to know what you want if you aren't properly communicating this!

Create realistic goals for yourself. Set a goal you think you could achieve, but then make the deadline one third longer than you originally wanted it. So, if you want to make $10,000 in three months, instead, make it four months. This way, you are more likely to get it done sooner and have a boost in your mood rather than failing to get it done at all.

Don't pin your emotional state on the expectation that you are hoping for. This is why disappointment is so hard to deal with. Your emotional state is what you experience in that moment. You can't wait to see how a situation unfolds to decide how you feel. Think about the example we discussed previously about inviting a friend to your party that sometimes flakes and sometimes shows up. You could base your mood on this outcome. If they show up, you are happy; if not, you are bummed to the point that your party is ruined. However, what you actually need to do is accept both outcomes. Know that if they come, that's great! If they don't, assure yourself that you will be satisfied either way.

[PART 3]
THINK FAST

[7]

HOW TO TRAIN YOUR BRAIN TO THINK FAST

There are close to 100 billion neurons in your brain. Can you even fathom how many that is? Even the richest men in the world have breached that 100 billion dollar mark within the past decade! There are more neurons in your brain than there are people in the world. This is an incredible potential that we don't fully recognize within our minds!

These neurons create connections within your brain, making this number even higher when you consider the new pairs consistently made. Each time you learn something new, a synapse is created between new neurons. The more that you know something, the better you remember it, the stronger the connection is going to be. This is why repetition is important for remembering things. It is like lifting weights. That first day you try to bench press 50 pounds, it is a struggle. After two weeks of doing this every day, it is easy! When you first meet someone, you might struggle to remember their names. After a week of getting to know them, there's no way you could forget who they are! That neuron is being worked out just like your biceps as you are lifting weights.

You have unlimited storage within your brain. Not only can you remember anything when you put your mind to it, but you can learn anything new with no limitation. Our brains have more storage than any laptop, phone, or other electronic devices we've ever had. You could read every book you've ever seen, watch every movie you've ever heard of, and meet every person living within a 50-mile radius of you and still have enough room in your brain to learn more. The more you know, the more you remember, and the easier it will be to learn new information. This is crucial to remember when we start to train our brains to think fast.

Trying to measure how much storage we have is nearly impossible, but we can make an estimate (Interlandi, 2016). It is estimated now that we have over 100,000 gigabytes of storage in our brains. We can't know if this is even the limit because no one has ever made it this high even when trying!

With all of this information we know now, it certainly lights a fire within us to learn as much as possible. The problem is, that can be challenging sometimes. We get distracted, confused, and flustered easily. What is it that keeps us from learning properly? Much of what we have discussed can get in the way, such as stress or procrastination. In this chapter, we're going to take a look at how you can start to think faster every day of your life. There are a few quick steps that you can take to think faster:

1. Relax to think clearly.
2. Look at the root of the problem.
3. Remove distractions.
4. Grow your mind to think quicker.

One challenging thing that might make it harder for you to think quickly is to think during times of stress and pressure. Let's discuss the how-to of thinking with mental tension.

How to Think Under Pressure and Stress

There are going to be times when you have to make a quick decision under an intense amount of stress or pressure. Maybe if you wait too late to decide you miss your chance, or perhaps someone else is trying to convince you to decide quicker. If you want to make informed decisions as often as possible, you'll have to train yourself to think under pressure and stress.

There are many dangers of overthinking that you have to be aware of. The reason that thinking in stressful times is so hard is that we think of all the worst possible scenarios. It is like a survival moment where our minds kick into survival mode to try and protect us from any potential dangers. If we don't know how to work through this mental blockage, then we won't be able to make a properly informed decision. The first thing that you will want to do when thinking under stress is to keep it minimal. As soon as you start thinking "What if?", cut your mind off because there are a lot of "what ifs" you could come up with. What if I make the wrong choice? What if I'm missing something important? What if I mess up big time? What if everyone dies? What if the world ends? You could make yourself sick with all of the what-ifs of the world!

We often struggle because we use personalization. We forget the different perspectives that others carry over the world and ourselves in general. You might immediately think, "Oh no, what am I going to do?" Remember the "we" involved in decisions. You are not alone even when it feels like you have no one you can count on.

The first thing that you will want to do when presented with a stressful situation is to remind yourself that you are not going to die. This is not the end of the world. This is not the worst thing that ever happened to you.

Take it one step at a time. Your mind will often jump to the end. You will only think about what might happen after the fact. Don't let this be the way you think! Start slow and take it one step at a time. Think of the "now" and then the next step and then the next step.

Sometimes, if you can't help but think of the end, consider what the worst possible outcome could be. What might happen that would make you think that this is it, this is the moment when it is all going downhill? Do your best to remain as positive as possible.

Don't feel so rushed. Oftentimes high-pressure situations can cause negative outcomes because we rush right through the important parts. Let's think of an example of a low-pressure situation so that you can understand how taking things slow is the best method to reduce stress in situations that demand urgency. You woke up late for work. You got ready in time, and if you leave now, you'll get to work five minutes late. However, you go to grab your car keys and they aren't there!

This is an immediate cause for concern. What if you can't find the keys? What if you're late for work? What if you get fired? What if someone broke into your house and stole your keys and stole your car? What if you never find your keys again? These are the thoughts that first pop into people's heads! The keys might be right behind you, but our brains can still take us to dark places when we get a little stressed.

What you would want to do in this situation is to stop and think. Freeze in the moment and don't think of anything other than what you did with your keys last. Where have you found them when you lost them before? Did you put them in a second popular spot for keys, wallets, etc.? Did you leave them in a purse or bag? Did you leave them in your pants pockets? Did you leave them in your car? Do you have house keys on them? Maybe they are sitting in your front door lock. Rather than jumping to those scary things ahead, stay focused on the moment and take it one step at a time.

How to Use Anchors and Physical Association

If you want to start to think faster, one method to improve this process is to use anchors. This is a physical object or touch that will help bring you to a mindset whenever you need to jump into that headspace.

This connects to high pressure because you could use an anchor as a stress reducer. One good anchor to start with is a small coin or stone that you can keep in your pocket. When you are feeling relaxed and in a positive mindset, hold this object. Touch it, feel it, and use it to remind yourself that even in your darkest moments, you have been able to get to this moment of peace afterward. When you are feeling stressed at work, out in public, or anywhere else, touch this object and have it anchor you back into a positive headspace.

To start anchoring, first, determine what the purpose of the physical association is going to be. If you want confidence, find something to hold onto for when you are giving a speech. When you start to choke up, you can touch this object to bring you to that confident place once again.

Use only positivity and confidence around this anchor to boost its powers. Your anchor could be something that you already carry with you, like a lipstick tube or a keychain. When you touch this anchor again, it is going to pull you right back into that mindset you had when creating this anchor.

You can start to use this on other people. It is a way to help you positively persuade others. One method is to use an anchor as leverage in a business meeting. Let's say that you're looking for investors and you're nervous about them agreeing to the deal you're presenting. At the beginning of the meeting, make everyone as happy as possible. Compliment them, give them a ton of smiles, and make sure everyone is taken care of. Before you start your speech or proposal, tap the table in front of you twice. Do it in a natural way, but touch the table in a way that is noticeable but not awkward. Give your speech or proposal, and once you're done, tap the table in the exact same way. You can, unknowingly to the listeners, anchor them and bring them back to that positive mood they were in when they arrived, heightening your chances of having a positive outcome.

[8]

IMPROVING DECISION-MAKING AND PROBLEM-SOLVING SKILLS

The worst thing that tarnishes our ability to make decisions is that we struggle because we are afraid of making the right one. In fact, the majority of the stress that we feel comes from being afraid that we might not be making the right one (Chen, Rossignac-Milon, & Higgins, 2018). Decision making isn't an easy process. This is why we often have others make the decision for us! Think of the last time that you went to the grocery store. Maybe you weren't sure what snack to buy. A display of candy bars or chips that were on sale helped make your decision. Then you got home and plopped in front of the TV, ready to find something good to watch. Rather than scrolling through, you went with the first pick of what was recommended for you. It felt like you made a decision, but most of these choices were made for you throughout the day.

When we struggle to make decisions, we struggle to problem solve as well. If you aren't sure of yourself, don't think critically, and have mental fog, then it will be hard to make a quick decision. Not all problems need instant solutions, but many of us still struggle to come up with the right answer because of all the other thoughts jumbled within our brain. In this chapter, we are going to give you the best decision-making and problem-solving methods so that you can think as fast as possible without letting these processes slow you down.

Making decisions can be hard because there's so much other fluff that can get in the way of clear thinking. Imagine that you are trying to make a cake in your kitchen. If stuff is cooking in the oven, there are dishes in the sink, and another person is trying to make a meal as well, it will be harder to focus on the cake! We have to keep a clear head in order to make it easier to think quickly. There are a few steps to do this:

1. Prioritize your thoughts.
2. Look at the most basic version of the problem or decision.
3. Conduct an analysis to find all possible options.

Let's first take a look at the how-to of prioritizing the most important thoughts.

How to Prioritize Important Thoughts

To work optimally and get the things done that need to be taken care of, you'll want to learn how to better prioritize the things that are most important to you. We often try and do the things that we want to get out of the way in that moment. Maybe you're cleaning your home and you have to do the dishes, do the laundry, and clean up your room. As you walk throughout the house, however, you see smaller tasks that need to get done, so it's easier to get distracted. What's most important, however, is that we prioritize the things that we initially wanted to get done as they are essential. You didn't think of completing the other tasks until they were right in front of you. So is it really all that important to you?

Sometimes everything seems like it is important. Your brain can be very good at convincing you of certain levels of urgency. Anything could be meaningless or dire if you thought about it.

If you have a problem or need to make a decision, there are some prioritization tools that you need. First, write a master list of everything needed to know about this situation. What needs to be done? What are the problems that are going to keep you from completing these tasks?

First, decide the level of importance, how quickly it needs to be done, and the estimated time that it will take to complete. Sometimes you will discover a problem that can be easily taken care of when you are able to prioritize properly.

It is essential that you narrow your options to the very core.

You won't be able to make the right decision if you aren't properly prioritizing your thoughts and actions.

Sometimes we struggle to make a decision because we are scared of what will happen if we don't make the right decision. We don't think about what that worst-case scenario is even going to be! Next, make sure to remind yourself to look at the past and discover that things turned out completely fine. You are OK today, so even when you made the wrong decision, everything ended up working out.

After this, use examples to help you make decisions. If you're really stuck, Google your specific question because someone online has likely had the same dilemma. Yahoo Answers, Reddit, and Quora are great user-based tools that many people use to share their struggles online. You can get multiple answers if you ever need more advice than what you are already experiencing.

The best decisions will be made when things are planned out, and you can't do this if you aren't properly planning in the first place! Sometimes we have to make sure that we plan before, rather than waiting until after we face the problem, to make the right decision.

How to Identify the Real Issue

One method for problem-solving is to look at the real issue that needs to be confronted. We often try to find solutions that will help get us out of a situation fast. You might want the quick fix or an easy alternative so that less effort is required. However, if you do try to take shortcuts, it can end up hindering your ability to find a positive solution in the end.

Sometimes, the person making the decision doesn't want to have to admit that they're wrong. Maybe it's a spouse, a boss, or someone else that refuses to accept responsibility for the outcome. What can you do to help get to the root of the issue? How can you find a solution without having to make them feel bad or prove them wrong in the first place?

It is important to train your brain to go directly to the core. Always ask "Why?" Go through the normal questions of who, what, where, when and why. Dig deeper and use your critical thinking skills to get you to the real problem that's hidden underneath it all. Think of the last time you had two friends fighting. They might have fought over something small, maybe one was rude to the other, or perhaps there was a little misunderstanding. Between two average individuals, maybe it's not a big deal, but these friends might have blown things out of proportion. Part of this is because there was likely a deeper issue hidden underneath the rest that made everything feel worse than what it was.

To understand how to make the best decisions and come up with the greatest solutions for certain problems, you can use a root-cause analysis. There are a few steps to this process. As an example, we are going to use the idea of someone that struggled to lose weight because the diets they have tried never worked.

First, identify what the issue is at face value. What is the most basic understanding of the problem? In our example, it is that someone struggles to lose weight.

Share this problem with someone else. Discuss it and gain a different perspective. In this example, the person that wants to lose weight might talk to a doctor, nutritionist, or even someone else that shares their struggles.

Look at all the things that could have caused or influenced this issue. This is when thinking becomes deeper. In this example, they struggle because they suffer from anxiety. Their mother was very hard on them about losing weight. They use food as a source of comfort. Exercising is difficult for them.

Come up with a few different solutions. At this point, you can see the many different causes; therefore, you can develop different solutions. In this example, you might talk to a professional about overcoming anxiety so the emotional eating stops, and they can work through issues with their mother. A better exercise routine can be presented as well.

Choose the solution that will work best. This would be dependent on the individual, but as you can see, the solutions that we came up with aren't simply "find a new diet plan" because that is not going to solve the root of the problem.

Decide if this was the right thing to do. After this analysis has happened and a solution is chosen, it's time to implement the strategy. The person trying to lose weight can see a therapist and sign up for a yoga class.

Fix and prepare anything else needed for this process. This is when you would reflect and determine if the best course of action had been taken. If weight loss is occurring, then the right solution was found. If no weight loss is happening, it's time to dig deeper or try out a new solution.

How to Use Reasoning, Judgment, Analysis, and Learning

Sometimes we want to find a solution to make the situation in front of us work. When we do this, we can quickly forget that there are alternatives available to us! Remember to start with reasoning. Don't look at things from your perspective. Consider all avenues of equal importance.

Next, you can form judgments. These judgments should be objective, but they can also be from your perspective. There are a few ways that you can improve your judgment skills. Make sure to recognize the faults of your past in order to pull valuable information that will keep you from repeating mistakes. You also have to recognize the biases that you experience. These include things such as:

1. your level of optimism/pessimism
2. how much you favor a person/place/idea
3. your expectancy of an event based on the probability that it has happened in the past
4. the ability to notice details/larger concepts

Make an analysis. Were you right / were you wrong? What needs adjusting? Here are your how-to steps of proper analysis:

1. Break it down into pieces to start with one area at a time.
2. Create a goal for what information you'd like to pull.
3. Gather all the important information needed.
4. Make judgments and correct the process to gain desired results.

Finally, you will take away something that you learned from this experience. Even in the most challenging scenarios, there will be something valuable that you can pull.

To increase your ability to do all of these things, you will have to research, practice, research, practice, and repeat over and over again. Practice is something that you have to do on your own, but let's take a look at some other methods of accelerated learning that can help drive your success even further.

[9]

HOW TO HACK YOUR WAY TO A SHARPER, SMARTER, FASTER, AND MORE RESILIENT BRAIN

For a long time, it was believed that our brains were static. Up until our mid-20s, our brains are constantly evolving. By the time we hit 30, it appeared for a while that we stopped growing. Many scientists thought that this also meant our brains couldn't change. It was believed that once you hit a certain age, you were the person that you are and there was no altering that.

Research has proven that this is not true anymore (Chapman, 2014). There are legitimate methods that you can use to "bio-hack" your way to a sharper mind. You can use your biology, not some outside source, to make your brain smarter and more resilient. You can think faster so that you are less likely to be influenced and can be free from the embarrassment of not feeling intelligent enough. You can learn anything you want as fast as your brain allows you, and this will help keep your mind ever-evolving. Let's look at the best methods and tips to make your learning speedier and more robust.

The best bio-hack tips that you can use are things that you can do with your mind! Here are a few things that you can use in order to think sharper, smarter, faster, and more resiliently:

1. Focus on your breathing through meditation and mindful activities.
2. Make sure your nutrition and physical health are in check.
3. Notice your heartbeat and count the rhythm to keep you focused on the present.
4. Change the lighting to make it dimmer when bright lights might be distracting.
5. Use a cold shower, step outside during winter, or hold an ice cube on your wrist for better concentration.

Let's look at some more extensive methods that you can use, along with a how-to description of the way that you can practically implement these methods into your life.

How to Accelerate Learning

Reading and writing is an important process in accelerated learning. You will want to practice doing research, taking notes, and writing your opinions to help you better understand the information that you're taking in.

Read what you are writing out loud. You will be able to discover anything about it that doesn't sound right when reading aloud. You will also have the ability to remember it better because you are repeating it, and you are learning it in a new way.

To become a better writer, just start writing! There is no secret, quick trick, or pill that you can take, which will magically make you a better writer. You will simply have to practice. You won't know what needs to be fixed or improved until you start to write and look back on what you created to discover a method for making it even greater.

Push past when you can't think of a word. If you are writing a sentence and you can't think of a better word, write it out and highlight or capitalize it. Then you can go back and check over these words or phrases and use a thesaurus to make it sound better.

To read faster, prep yourself by skimming the entire text. Take note of headlines, look over pictures, get a glimpse of graphs, and give yourself a sense of what you need to emphasize as you are reading.

If you read something and feel like you need to go back to it, don't. This is often a trick in our brain that makes us think we need to research further. Just keep reading!

Stop the subvocalizing in your head from keeping you

reading slower. This is a process in which your brain tries to say out loud the things that you're reading. Silence this by distracting yourself. You can chew gum when reading, fidget with something in your hand, or use a bookmark to underline the words as you're reading through.

Read the first sentence of every paragraph of a text if you really want to be a speedy reader. Most of the time, the remainder of a paragraph is further explanation to the point that was initially made at the beginning of the paragraph. The final sentence is usually one that wraps it up as well and helps to transition to the next point.

This is something else that you will have to continually practice. The faster and more frequently you read, the faster and better you will be at reading later on. This is important because when you are reading something online, there are usually many hyperlinks hidden. These are blue or underlined words that take you to a different page. You should be reading these because they are often the source of information. When you can read the article and all of its sources, you can better form your opinion rather than basing your views on what the writer of the article said.

This is a process that you need to remember to enjoy. There is nothing good that's going to come from torturing yourself! Learning is a privilege and it should be something that you accept wholeheartedly.

If you don't understand, then look for a new way to learn certain bits of information. If you're reading a book and it doesn't make any sense, try seeing if there's a video on it and vice versa.

How to Avoid the Biggest Issues When Brain Training

The biggest issue that people have when training their brain is thinking that they already know enough. Never limit yourself and always look for new chances to learn information.

Don't be afraid of failure. The biggest failure you could make is failing to do anything at all. Another mistake that people make is that they don't understand the things that they're learning. If you can't explain it down to its deepest core, then you don't understand it! You should be able to take the things you know and teach them to someone else.

Forget about memorization that doesn't do you any good. Memorization is for playing games, not for operating through life. When you truly know something and understand it, that will take you farther than knowing the names or dates of something you're trying to memorize.

If you don't understand something, explain it like you would to a five-year-old. How would you tell this information to a child that is hearing about it for the first time? What ways could you explain something to an alien if they were to ask you about the topic you're studying?

Stop making excuses. There is always a new way and a new solution to go about things. There is nothing that is unachievable when you start to learn. No information is too hard to learn, and nothing that you learn about will be useless even if you can't practically apply it.

Challenge yourself. Too many people are afraid of a challenge. They think it'll be painful. Embrace these struggles. If your challenges are continuously no fun, then you should look for a new way to go about them.

How to Use Brain Integration

We have a big brain in our skulls, but most of the time, people only use a portion of their brain. Your brain has two sides, as we discussed previously. In order to incorporate your brain even more, you need to start to look for ways for brain integration. This is when you bring both sides of your brain together, are able to connect mentality to physicality, and when you have the chance to use as much of your brain as possible.

When learning information, remember to associate it with the visuals around you. Always look for brain integration activities. These are things that are going to be visual, logical, creative, and mental. This is different from multitasking. Rather, it is a task that has multiple purposes.

Singing and dancing at the same time can be one. This makes you think about your body, your voice, and your thoughts as you move around the house or change your voice to match a tune.

Do something simple like rubbing your head and patting

your belly at the same time. This can be enough to lock both sides of your brain together!

Cooking is a great way to keep your brain integrated. Cleaning is another method that can keep your mind focused. They present you with tasks that you have to come up with a solution for. Look for innovative ways to do these things, especially when they start to feel mundane.

Other brain integration activities include:

- gardening
- standing while reading
- exercising with a machine
- playing an instrument
- logical games and puzzles
- video games

The more that you challenge your brain, the more you are setting yourself up for success!

[PART 4]
PRACTICE

21 NEUROSCIENCE WAYS TO THINK CLEAR AND FAST

We've given you methods and strategies to rewire your brain throughout this book, but now we are going to give you actual practical exercises, with tips and tricks to help make your brain as efficient as possible.

#1 – TRY THE PINKY AND THUMB INTEGRATION TECHNIQUE.

As we previously mentioned, brain integration is an important part of increasing your overall neurological powers. One method of brain integration that you can try frequently is the pinky and thumb game. Whenever you are feeling anxious, stressed, lost in the moment, mentally cluttered, and so on, you can use this technique to pull you back to the present and get both sides of your brain working hard. To play, make a fist with each hand and hold them out in front of you. With your left hand, stick your pinky out. With your right hand, stick your thumb out. Count to three, and on three, swap the positions that your hands are in. This would mean sticking out your left thumb and right pinky. It is a lot harder than you'd think! The trick is to do it in an instant, both hands swapping at the same time. The first few times you try, you might find that you end up sticking out both your pink and thumb at the same time!

#2 – PLAY THE 5 "WHY?" GAME.

Whenever you learn something new, have to question a theory, or generally need a solution to something that might be stressing you or causing worry, play the 5 "Why?" game. This requires you to ask "why" five levels deep. Anyone who has a child knows that this is a common game that toddlers like to play! You will tell them something and then they have to ask "why" until both of you are exhausted! You can do it with anything. Next time you learn something new, ask "Why?" about it at least five times. If you learned that your brain reacts poorly to stress, ask why? You discover it is because stress increases certain hormones. Why? These hormones are a response to stress so that you are prepared for outside threats. Why? We have a natural defense mechanism within us for survival. Why? All living things have their defense mechanisms, it is natural. Why? This is the question that will be the hardest! Usually by the time you get to the fifth "Why?" you've reached something existential which only you can discover the conclusion!

#3 - TAKE A DIFFERENT ROUTE TO WORK.

Every day, we do the same thing in a certain way. Even if your job requires random hours, an unsteady schedule, or something else that causes a lot of variation, there are still plenty of rituals that we participate in that we don't even notice. Your brain can easily go on autopilot when you are not paying attention. If we do everything ritualistically, eventually our brain stops being challenged, decreasing our cognitive abilities. Rather than letting this be the case, do your best to look for small ways to switch up your routine. This is going to help you stay clear and focused throughout your day. Take the long way to work, switch up your route, and look for other methods of taking a different way to work.

#4 - THINK OF YOUR ANXIETY LIKE AN UNWANTED HOUSE GUEST.

Anxiety and stress are going to be the biggest mood killers. It is like dropping a bucket of paint on a beautiful portrait! To help alleviate your anxiety, picture it as a houseguest that you are kicking out! They have stayed on your couch for far too long, always nagging and making you scared. It is time to kick them out! Whenever you hear that anxiety or stress knocking, slam the door in their face! Every once in awhile, you might still see them on the street, and they'll have something to shout at you. Whatever you do, don't let them back in your home! This is the way you can think of anxiety.

When you get those creeping thoughts like, "What if everyone hates me? What if the worst possible situation happens?", slam the door! This type of visualization makes it easier to recognize and manage your emotional state.

#5 – ORGANIZE WITH YOUR EYES CLOSED.

This sounds pretty counterintuitive! How could one possibly organize if their eyes are closed? This is going to be helpful because it forces you to use clues not related to sight in order to organize. Find something small that needs to be organized. Maybe it is your sock drawer or some change that you want to sort out. Sit down somewhere comfortable, dump out the contents of what needs to be organized in front of you, and sort it as best as you can without peeking. Afterward, you can adjust and fix anything you messed up, but you might be surprised by your abilities! If you have a bucket of change that you want to sort, you will have to feel the weight and texture of the coins to determine which is which. If you are sorting socks, you'll have to feel their length, softness, and thickness to determine whether or not they might be a match. There are plenty of small forms of organization your home could probably use, so try to do it without looking to increase cognitive function!

#6 - EXPLAIN YOUR SITUATION FROM A DIFFERENT PERSPECTIVE.

When you have a problem that you need to solve on your own, it can be challenging to sometimes come up with our solutions. This is partly because we don't have the right perspective. If you are stuck at the bottom of a well, your only option is to try and claw your way out. Those outside the well are going to have a much better perspective on what to do to help pull you from this place. When you have a problem, pretend as though one of your friends is currently going through the situation that you are in. How might you comfort them? What would you tell them to help that person find clarity or understand deeper what it is that they're going through? What tools could you provide to them to work through the challenging scenario? By stepping outside your own life for a moment and picturing that you are in someone else's, not only are you gaining a perspective that gives you clarity, but you also understand what you are going through with a different mentality entirely. Your problem might not seem so big, you might discover that it is more of a blessing than a curse, and so on.

#7 - TRY THE POMODORO TECHNIQUE.

Studies have proven that your brain learns better in shorter periods of time (Saez, n.d.). Rather than sitting there for six hours to study, and then taking an hour-long break, this suggests that you take shorter breaks frequently. When an hour begins, you work for twenty-five minutes, take a break for five, work again for twenty-five minutes, and then a final break. You would repeat this process as needed as you are studying or working. The reason this works is that your brain is willing to be committed for those twenty-five minutes. That's enough time to stay in focus, and the promise of the break is good to keep you going. If you have to study for four hours and you look ahead and think about that big chunk of time, it is harder to find the motivation because it seems like such a daunting task. Breaking it up is easier to manage and helps enable you to stick to the process.

#8 – BRUSH YOUR TEETH WITH THE OPPOSITE HAND.

Another integral brain exercise is to switch the hand that you use to brush your teeth. We have a dominant hand and that can create a dominant side. In order to work out all aspects of your body, it is important that you use both sides of your body when possible. You can't always write with the opposite hand, as this is something that we have to practice doing from a young age! You can learn how to do other simple tasks with the opposite hand, like brushing your teeth. After trying this and swapping out hands for several weeks, start to try harder things. Cook, clean, and scroll your phone with the opposite hand. You'll be surprised at how much this simple task can change your overall brainpower!

#9 - WATCH SOMETHING THAT YOU DON'T LIKE.

In school, we were forced to do all kinds of things we didn't like. Maybe you were a science kid that only wanted to learn about space, but you still had to sit in history class. Perhaps you were athletic and hated having to sit through drawing. However, these lessons still taught you something, and there was valuable information discovered that's still relevant to your life today. If you were in charge of your curriculum the entire time, it would have severely limited the amount of information that you would have been able to take in. We've stopped exposing ourselves to things we don't like, and there is a lot to be learned from entertainment and information outside our comfort zone. Whatever it is that you don't enjoy, whether it is action movies, documentaries, dramas, and so on, try something that you wouldn't normally watch. Even if you dislike it, find something to be learned from what you are viewing.

#10 - COOK SOMETHING YOU'VE NEVER EATEN.

Cooking frequently can help you stay more focused. It is a mindful activity that requires you to pay attention the entire time. You have to come up with a plan, work to execute that plan, and reflect on the results that you've been given. It is an important process that helps your cognition. Take it a step further by cooking something that you never have before. Better yet, cook something you haven't even eaten! A meat type of might be scary since you could undercook it if not done properly. However, try something low risk and experiment. Create your own recipe! When you eat this food for the first time, you won't compare it to something else, helping your esteem as well.

#11 – PLAN OUT WHAT YOUR MESS WILL LOOK LIKE AFTER YOU'VE CLEANED.

Sometimes it is hard to tackle a big messy project. Maybe your office desk looks like a paper printing company. Perhaps it is the garage that has half-finished projects and tools strewn throughout. Does your closet look like a rampaged retail store? Wherever your biggest mess might be that you want to improve on, visualize what it will look like once you have managed to do all the cleaning. This is going to be the perfect method to make it easier to tackle your biggest messes. The reason why we sometimes struggle to complete a project is that we can't fathom what it will look like once done. If we don't believe that something is possible, then we don't know how to put in the effort to complete that. When you are feeling overwhelmed with the completion of a project, remember to visualize what it will look like. Stand in front of that messy desk and picture how it will look once clean. It seems so simple, but you will be surprised at how much this will help you work through your messiest spaces.

#12 - READ AN ENTIRE BOOK OUT LOUD.

You have the ability to read much faster than you can talk. Try reading this sentence and then try saying it out loud. When you read a word like "saying," in your brain, it is a quick instance. Speaking, it takes longer since there are two syllables. Pick a book, something on the shorter side, but do your best to read this out loud throughout a week or so. It is going to take you a lot longer to finish the book, but you will discover that you comprehend it much more. You will probably be able to recall certain moments easier, and you might notice some things that you didn't if you have already read this book of choice. You have to take longer to read the book and understand each word. Sometimes when we're reading, we might not even know what a word means, but continue through because it is easier to comprehend meaning through context. If you have to say it out loud, then you are forcing yourself to learn this new word, what it means, and how it sounds. After this activity, you will start to discover how much easier it is for you to understand and remember information when you take longer to comprehend.

#13 - ASSOCIATE WHAT YOU ARE LEARNING WITH A PLACE YOU KNOW.

If you are trying to study for a test that requires you to remember a lot of information, it can be daunting to think about your ability to remember it all. One method to make it easier for you to remember information is to associate it with a place that you are familiar with. You can choose an entire home, or you might visualize a small space, like a desk or a kitchen cabinet. Let's use the example of learning the planets in order. This is basic knowledge that not many would struggle to remember in their adult years, but it is still a good example of how you can use this method for learning. The order of the planets is Mercury, Venus, Earth, Mars, Jupiter, Saturn, Uranus, and Neptune. Let's say that you choose your home as the visual space. You walk in the door, and the first room you are in is the kitchen. As you walk through the house, you pass a bathroom, your roommate's bedroom, the living room, your room, your bathroom, the basement, the dining room, and then the door to the backyard. You would then associate the first bathroom with Mercury. Your roommate's bedroom is Venus. The living room is Earth. Your room is Mars. Your bathroom is Jupiter. The basement is Saturn and the dining room is Uranus. When you can't remember the order, you can remember the path through your house and which planet is associated with which room to give you a better chance at retaining this information!

#14 - DRAW A MAP OF A PLACE YOU WANT TO RECALL.

We have a lot more stored in our memory that we give our brains credit for. Have you ever cleaned out a room and as you are going through things, you discover items that you completely forgot you had? You simply forgot for a moment,

but that item you found not only sparked your remem-
brance over the possession of this object, but you also start
to remember all the other past situations involving this thing.
If you can create visual clues and other monumental
anchors associated with a memory, it can help you to
uncover more that you had forgotten. Pick a time in your life
that you wish you could remember more of. Maybe it is your
college days, the time when you lived on a farm when you
were 5 years old, or maybe it is even something as simple as
a vacation last year. Pick a place from this time period and
draw a map from memory. You can do a simple blueprint
like a bird's-eye view of the rooms of a house. You could get
more complex and create a map of the entire neighborhood
you grew up in. As you are recreating this past place, you
will start to recall more and more about each place that a
memory was created. You will uncover things that you
forgot you even had stored in that noggin of yours. After
you've completed this task, try doing something even
further. Color in the map, make it more detailed, map out
the furniture in a room, and so on. After trying from
memory, look at old pictures or actual maps to fill in any
holes you don't quite remember.

#15 - REACT USING YOUR FACIAL FEATURES ONLY.

To think faster and clearer, we have to better understand our
emotions so that nothing gets in the way of our cognition.
We have to have a better understanding of different types of
language and the way in which we communicate with each

other. One activity you can do to increase your ability to understand and express body language is to react using your facial features only. Practice alone in front of a mirror first. What would your face look like if you heard something shocking? How might you react if you were angry? If you wanted to let someone know that you were happy, what face would you make? After you've recognized these facial features, start to get a little more complex. What face would you make to let others know that you support them? How would you show disappointment? When you are more aware of your body language, you will be more aware of how you can control this in the settings needed to get your desired outcome as well. You can express yourself better to show your true feelings, and you will set yourself up for success.

#16 - TURN OFF YOUR PHONE FOR A DAY.

This sounds scary for some! How could you go an entire day without a phone? If you aren't an emergency room doctor on call or even a parent that's away from their child, you have no reason to leave your phone on all day! A friend might text you, maybe you get a work email, or perhaps your mother tries to call. These things can usually wait a day. If you are that desired of a person that others will worry when you don't answer, make a social media post or send a text to your closest friends to let them know you are shutting out the online world for a day. Start with a six-hour block if an entire day is too scary for you. The first thing you will notice is how anxious you might feel that you are missing out on something. Remember that most of the time, you are not getting constant texts and calls anyway! The next thing you will discover is that you have to find satisfaction from outside sources. If you are sitting there bored on the train, you might reach for your phone, but on this blackout day, you will have to entertain yourself by reading a book or staring out the window. You will start to notice that you have to figure things out for yourself more. Maybe you want to Google something, but instead, you'll have to try and figure it out on your own. Phones are incredibly important to how society operates, and it is fine to use your phone frequently. What we have to understand to think faster, clearer, and more critically is how dependent we are on technology. Don't think you have to toss your phone forever, but make yourself aware of how crucial this little electronic device is in your life. The more dependent you are on it, the less you are thinking on your own, and that's an important skill we don't want to lose.

#17 – PAINT A PICTURE FROM MEMORY ONLY.

This is similar to the activity involving the memory map, only a little more detailed. It also doesn't have to be a picture of a scene from your memory either. You can look up a picture online or find an old one in your phone. Whatever it is, pick out a picture that you think you could either draw or paint easily, based on your artistic skills. For example, if you are a terrible artist and struggle to even draw a square without making it look weird, a picture of a detailed pasture with flowers, trees, clouds, and animals shouldn't be your top pick. Find your picture and pick your artistic medium. You could use a canvas and paint, or simply use a pencil and a piece of paper. Recreate the image of choice as detailed as you can using only your memory. Avoid going back to it as a reference throughout the activity to ensure that you are doing your best to force your memory to work in overdrive. After you've completed the picture, you can make a comparison. If it is way different, try again! Or you can move on and pick a different picture. The point of this will be for you to study what's important beforehand as you collect all the information on the image needed to finish it properly. Then, as you are painting or drawing, you'll need to use context clues and figure out what the picture looked like. When you make the comparison of what you did versus what the actual image was, it gives you the chance to understand your strengths and weaknesses about memory and understanding an image.

#18 - FORCE LAUGHTER EVERY DAY FOR A WEEK AND KEEP TRACK OF HOW YOU FEEL.

A huge part of learning is being in the right mindset to do so. If you can improve your mood more frequently and stay mindful in that moment, it will be easier to remember the things you experience. Rather than wasting mental energy on stress and anxiety, you can find use from these emotions and keep a positive mindset that helps you grow and learn throughout your life. An activity that can drastically help your mood is to force laughter. Just smiling at yourself in the mirror can sometimes be enough to turn your mood around. Start by doing this throughout your day and notice how it makes you feel. Then, every day for a week, force yourself to laugh for at least a minute. It is a 60-second exercise done seven times, and you will see great results. Write down in a journal your mood every day and give your happiness/anger a rating on a 1-10 scale. The results after this week is over might shock you!

#19 – REPHRASE SOMETHING TO MAKE IT SOUND LIKE THE OPPOSITE.

A lot of what we learn and how we comprehend has to do with perspective. You see things through your eyes, and others do the same. This means that we can take one situation and turn it into whatever fits our perspective. In order to help you understand this, take the happiest moment of your life and one of the biggest personal struggles that you have had. Imagine that your happy moment is like a comedy and the worst a drama. How could you take those two movies, but turn them into the opposite? Could that good memory be someone else's nightmare? Is your struggle someone else's comedy? The more you understand perspective, the easier it will be to comprehend the actual reality of the situation rather than a created perspective.

#20 – WATCH A MOVIE YOU'VE SEEN WITH THE CAPTIONS ON.

Movies are all about having big popular actors, exciting scenes, expensive costumes, and so on. A big part of understanding the story, however, lies within the dialogue. After you've watched a movie, you know what happened, the major plot points, and any spoilers. For this activity, the purpose is going to be to help you better understand what that actual movie means. What is the story behind it, and what is the message that's trying to be sent? When you read dialogue that you already know, you won't be focused on what's going to happen next. This is a comprehension exercise to help you understand the deeper meaning behind something that you are already aware of. There are likely noises, sentences, and other parts of the audio that will be discovered which you didn't pick up on the first time around. Give yourself this opportunity to discover greater meaning underneath.

#21 – LIMIT A SENSE FOR A DAY.

Most are born with five senses--sight, hearing, smell, taste, and touch. Not everyone still has these five senses, but for many of us, we use these without thinking much about it. For a day or a large period of time when you don't have much to do, pick a sense and limit this. Of course, we can think about "what if we couldn't see/hear/touch/smell," and so on. You might envision what it is like, but that's much different than experiencing that. We take these senses for granted, and we don't always comprehend how much they play in our overall cognition. Wear earplugs for an entire day or wear a blindfold or eye patch. You can limit your taste and smell too, but it is more challenging, so cutting back on your hearing or sight is a good first pic! Make sure that you won't hurt yourself, but experiment with your senses and discover how crucial they are for your learning.

BONUS. 20 MEMORY IMPROVEMENT EXERCISES

If you find that you are forgetting a lot of things, you might be greatly disturbed by it. But you don't have to feel that you are helpless, because you can keep your brain healthy and you can improve its overall state.

A study in the journal *Neurology* talks about how older Americans who physically exercise their bodies every day are likely to be less affected by neurological disorders, which cause memory loss and limited mobility. On the other hand, people who engage in physical activity may be able to keep their brains strong and healthy and also reduce the risk of cognitive impairment. Let's now look at some brain exercises you can do every day to keep your memory sharp and healthy.

Exercises to Sharpen Your Memory

1. Drive or Follow a New Route Home

It may seem trite and straightforward, but following a new route home will do wonders for your brain. If you get out of the routine movements of your life, your senses will be forced to discover the way home, which keeps your mind moving. Then you won't mindlessly go through the motions of going home without any reflection or consideration. You should avoid getting bored or putting your brain on auto-pilot. Mindless routines can cause us to get stuck and unable to move forward. Therefore, it is crucial to find ways to improve our overall mental state. Driving or walking home in a new way is going to give a boost to your mental sharpness.

2. Repeat Something Aloud

If you want to remember anything that you have just read, heard, or done, try repeating it aloud. For example, you might be talking to someone for the first time. You introduce yourself to him or her and then repeat his or her name. When you do that, you will be able to remember their name in no time. This also goes for reading. Often, it takes reading something aloud for us to commit it to memory. Sometimes, talking briefly out loud to yourself can be a helpful tool in enabling you to do all the things you want to do. Try doing that. It will save you a lot of hassle, and you might just be able to remember more things.

3. Listen to a Text While You Read

This method has been proven to help second language learners as they are reading a book in another language. You can try reading something to yourself silently in your native language while simultaneously listening to it read in the target language. When you use this method, you will engage your senses more and enable your mind to remember things a lot better. You can also do this with simple texts, as well. If you read along as someone else reads the version with you, then you will likely remember more from the text, because you will have engaged your listening and reading skills.

4. Play Crossword Puzzles

One way that many people improve their memory is by playing word games and crossword puzzles. Games like Scrabble where you can rearrange letters and make many words will enable your brain to think more clearly and you will be able to remember more. There is a reason why your grandparents would always do this. It is because when you play crossword puzzles, you allow yourself to assemble the words and concepts in your mind, which creates a vivid picture that will help you remember things better. Word games strengthen your vocabulary and enable you to do many things.

5. Play Chess

In addition to word games, don't forget to play games like

chess and checkers, because these games are strategy-based. When you play these games, you use your logical reasoning and strategy to master different situations. Additionally, you will feel more confident to handle all the things you need to do.

6. Learn to Play a Musical Instrument

Next, start to play a musical instrument. When you play an instrument like a violin or piano, you can engage the senses and remember something for a long time. Playing an instrument is also going to strengthen many of your other skills, including academics. It has been shown that playing a musical instrument can help a student get higher grades in school, which helps them greatly. It also makes a person well-rounded, because they feel they can do all things well. It's a great confidence booster. Plus, just knowing different composers can be useful, as you can access the knowledge of music wherever you go. Music contributes to our mind's ability to concentrate more intently on things, as well. Study with a teacher. Join a band or orchestra. Do whatever it takes to make some music. You won't regret it for an instant.

7. Play a Sport

Some people like to play individual sports, while others like to do team sports. It all depends on the person, and you should do whatever suits you. Try a sport that builds your confidence and helps you to focus. If you're into individual sports, then try swimming or running. If you want to join a team, play basketball or some similar sport. It will help you improve your concentration. Athletic exercise helps improve both your physical health and your mental health. When you sweat at the gym, you will feel the effects both in your body and mind.

8. Learn a Foreign Language

Learning a foreign language enriches the mind deeply. The brainpower of a bilingual person is very powerful. When you can think about concepts in two or more languages, you are using your brain in a comprehensive way that maximizes its ability. Learning a foreign language is a fun thing, too. It can be easier than many think, and you can experience greater freedom than ever before because you can access other cultures through language. Besides, you can make more friends from different nationalities. When you learn a foreign language, you build your vocabulary and enable your mind to absorb the sights and sounds of a culture. This helps you to remember concepts and ideas in a more organized way. It challenges you to think outside the box and **experience new things. It is a win-win.**

9. Draw a Map of an Area from Memory

After visiting a new place, you can challenge your mind to remember by drawing a map of the place. Often, our brains capture images that can be remembered for ages to come. Once you return from visiting a place, you can remember all the sights and sounds of that place, which will help you continually be mindful of it. Also, you can draw pictures of your daily life, including your commute, neighborhood, and other parts of your routine, which will enhance your mind and develop your memory.

10. Learn How to Make a New Dish

Cooking is a skill that can be mastered by almost anyone and it doesn't take too much effort. You can also take a cooking class to learn how to master a unique cuisine. When you cook, you stimulate different areas of the brain, which are associated with the senses, including smell, taste, and sight. Cooking can be a fun way to meet new people. Plus, you can enjoy the comforts of the food right at home. You won't have to go anywhere. Instead, you can have a great time cooking and make amazing dishes. You can also challenge yourself by trying out various new recipes. Then, you won't be making the same thing over and over mindlessly. Instead, you allow your brain to try out new things. It's important to give your brain a boost. You won't regret it for an instant.

11. Try Doing Your Chores with Your Eyes Closed

Instead of always doing your chores with your eyes open, try to do them eyes closed. For example, you could wash the dishes, fold your laundry, or even take a shower with your eyes closed. When you do this, you will require your brain to use alternate ways to get the task done. However, you should not do anything with your eyes closed that could be dangerous to you or other people.

12. Eat Your Food with Chopsticks

We are all used to eating food with a fork and knife in the United States. It makes for an easy meal to eat. However, not every culture uses a fork and a knife. If you go to an Asian country, you may find yourself requesting a fork, but they often won't have them on hand. Therefore, learning to use chopsticks is a must. When you use chopsticks, you will activate your brain and enable it to do motor skills that you may have never used before. It is a helpful exercise for you. In addition to being challenging to your brain, it also helps you to be culturally sensitive and aware. Then, you can eat with chopsticks anywhere with any meal, especially in Asia. It's a great thing both mentally and culturally. Challenge yourself to use chopsticks today. When you order take-out from a Chinese restaurant, request chopsticks. You won't regret it.

13. Use Your Non-Dominant Hand Sometimes

We get used to using our dominant hands for any kind of function, whether that is brushing our teeth or eating with a fork. However, if you want to challenge yourself more, try using your non-dominant hand. It can be a bit hard at first, but then you will see how you can effectively train yourself to do this.

14. Meet New People

One way that you can enhance your memory is by meeting new people. When you meet a new person, you stimulate your brain and develop new ideas about the world. For some people, especially introverts, this task can be daunting. Some have trouble with names and faces and are therefore quite shy when around new people. However, if you can challenge yourself to meet and get to know more new people, you will feel more confident and able to engage with new ways of thinking. Widening your social circle will help you to have more friends, contacts, and people with whom you can find something in common. It helps bring you together with people who might be unlike you but could be very good to have as friends or acquaintances. Don't limit yourself only to your social circle. Try to break out sometimes and meet new people. You will find people to be much more helpful and interesting. And in some cases, you might meet a friend for life.

15. Practice Mindful Eating

Another thing you can do is practice mindful eating. This means savoring each and every meal you have. Identify the different ingredients in your food, including spices, salt, and other tastes. When you mentally go through the process of tasting and experiencing the food, then you will enjoy your meal more. Plus, you will be a more "live to eat" kind of person, rather than "eat to live." It helps to be someone who greatly appreciates food. That is what makes life worth living. When you go to a restaurant alone or with other people, take time to taste the food genuinely. Allow your taste buds to absorb the flavors and be mindful of every bite you take. You may feel like you're always in a hurry, but you should slow down sometimes and enjoy the moment. It will feel a little bit awkward at first because we live in such a fast-paced culture. But you can do it!

16. Try to Do Math Problems in Your Head

In today's world, we're often rushing to the calculator and use a pen or pencil to find out the answers to math problems. But if you want to help yourself remember better, try doing them in your head. Better yet, do it while walking or some other physical activity. When you can multitask and give yourself more time to do it, you will find that it will strengthen you and give you more mental energy.

17. Practice Meditation

Sometimes we need to be quiet and concentrate our minds on softness. With our world that cannot stop talking, we need to have the space to be quiet and meditate. When you sit in silence and allow yourself to be mindful of your surroundings, then you will feel much better about things in your life. Benefits of meditation include stress relief, improved concentration, memory enhancement, and the reversal of cognitive decline. Meditation has a place in your life. You don't necessarily have to be sitting down, Indian-style on a yoga mat. It can be writing things down, taking a walk, or finding other ways to let out stress. Practicing meditation can greatly enhance your life. You will be able to handle all different kinds of situations, and you will be able to conquer the negative emotions in your life.

A crucial complement to meditation is having a positive

mindset. It's always important to be positive in whatever situation you face. Sometimes we act in negative ways, and we might also be caught up by many negative emotions, but we have to stop ourselves from flying off the handle. When you meditate or spend time praying or doing other related activities, you will feel much better and more relaxed. Then, you will be able to tackle any challenge you may face in your life.

18. Memorize Phone Numbers and Other Figures

You can strengthen your memory by memorizing the phone numbers and names of people in your life. It will be an important difference you can experience. Often, we can divide 10-digit numbers into smaller sections, enabling you to remember better. If you break them up into groups of three or four, then you will know the number well. For example, try memorizing the number 222 435 7890. It is easier to remember when you group it that way than it is for you to remember 2224357890. When our brain sees large figures, we might easily be overwhelmed. However, when we break things up into chunks, then our brains can process the information faster and more efficiently.

19. Do Arts and Crafts

Crafts, such as drawing, painting or knitting are becoming more popular, because they can boost our brainpower. Whenever you take up one of these hobbies, you will strengthen your fine motor skills and enable your brain to think more effectively. Doing a craft allows us to think creatively. When you are creative, then you allow your mind to think freely and out of the box. You are no longer confined to simple things. Instead, you can strengthen your mind's ability to reason and do other activities. Be creative. Draw a picture or paint on a canvas. You will find yourself expanding your range of possibilities. Use your imagination. You can do it!

20. Tell Stories and Recite Poetry

Telling a story is one of the most important ways you can remember information. It helps you to remember all different kinds of things in your life clearly. You can also recite a poem by heart. When you do this, you will be memorizing not just the words but how to pronounce them. It will greatly improve your cognitive functions. It can also help improve your life, if you or a loved one is struggling with Alzheimer's disease or dementia. It can mitigate the effects of neurological disorders, which can be challenging to live with. Therefore, find ways of integrating the recitation of stories and poetry in your routine, and you will find yourself able to do more things.

CONCLUSION

You can do so much with your hands, your body, your face, and every other part that makes you the person you are. The most powerful thing in your body exists within your head. Your brain is an incredibly powerful organ that will never fail to amaze even the most talented scientists out there. The problem is that it isn't thinking in the way that you want it to. Your brain can get hung up on small details, become easily distracted, and forget important information that you want to remember.

The solution is to incorporate methods of thinking clearly, thinking critically, and thinking fast. When you practice applying these methods and practical tips that have been discussed throughout this book, you are unlocking your greatest potential.

If you want to think fast and think critically, then it all starts with learning how to think clearly. There are many things that can cloud your mind. Stress, distractions, memories, regret, guilt, and other thoughts that pass through our brain can make it difficult to understand what it is that is going on up in that skull of yours. The better that we equip ourselves with the tools needed to understand our mind, the happier and healthier life we will be able to live. Many individuals will go throughout their life with high potential but are never able to follow through with that. This is because they aren't giving themselves the chance to think as efficiently as possible.

Once you start to clear up your thought processes, it becomes easier to start to think critically. This is the type of thought that will set you apart from everyone else. Those who can think critically can achieve anything they put their mind to. If you know how to investigate, analyze, and do the proper research on everything that you care about learning in your life, you are setting yourself up for success. The more critically you think, the easier it is to make better choices, avoid mistakes, and prevent yourself from falling into certain mental traps.

The benefit of both clear thinking and critical thoughts is that you will have a more resilient brain. It will be easier to think fast because you have set yourself up to learn as much information as possible within a shorter period. You will be smarter than others because you can consume a large amount of information within a shorter time. You can set yourself up to read faster, accelerate your learning, and think more logically in the end.

If there is one thing that you take away from this book and one thing only, it should be that there is no limit on your mind. Of course, there are limits on the things you can do in this world. You can't hurt others, you can't always get what you want, and you can't always change the minds of people around you. One thing that you will always be able to do, no matter what other aspects in your life might restrict you or create boundaries, will be the ability to change the way that you think. Always look for ways to grow, never limit your potential, and think freely and critically whenever you get the chance.

REFERENCES

Bregman, P. (2010). How and why to stop multitasking. Retrieved from https://hbr.org/2010/05/how-and-why-to-stop-multitaski

Chapman, S. (2014). 7 secrets to turbocharging your brain. Retrieved from https://www.psychologytoday.com/us/blog/make-your-brain-smarter/201412/7-secrets-turbocharging-your-brain

Chen, C. Y., Rossignac-Milon, M., & Higgins, E. T. (2018, February 12). Feeling distressed from making decisions: Assessors' need to be right. *Journal of Personality and Social Psychology*. Advance online publication. http://dx.doi.org/10.1037/pspp0000181

Cherry, K. (2019). How hindsight bias affects how we view

the past. Retrieved from https://www.verywellmind.com/what-is-a-hindsight-bias-2795236

Hasenkamp, W. (2013). How to focus a wandering mind. Retrieved from https://greatergood.berkeley.edu/article/item/how_to_focus_a_wandering_mind

Hershfield H. E. (2011). Future self-continuity: How conceptions of the future self transform intertemporal choice. Retrieved from https://www.ncbi.nlm.nih.gov/pmc/articles/PMC3764505/

Interlandi, J. (2016). New estimate boosts the human brain's memory capacity 10-fold. Retrieved from https://www.scientificamerican.com/article/new-estimate-boosts-the-human-brain-s-memory-capacity-10-fold/

Michl, L. C., McLaughlin, K. A., Shepherd, K., & Nolen-Hoeksema, S. (2013). Rumination as a mechanism linking stressful life events to symptoms of depression and anxiety: Longitudinal evidence in early adolescents and adults. Retrieved from https://www.ncbi.nlm.nih.gov/pmc/articles/PMC4116082/

Psychologist World. (n.d.) Psychology of choice. Retrieved from https://www.psychologistworld.com/cognitive/choice-theory#references

Pychyl, T. (2018). The neural signature of procrastination. Retrieved from https://www.psychologytoday.com/us/blog/dont-delay/201808/the-neural-signature-procrastination

Saez, F. (n.d.). The science behind the pomodoro technique. Retrieved from https://facilethings.com/blog/en/science-behind-pomodoro-technique

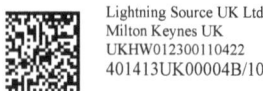

Lightning Source UK Ltd.
Milton Keynes UK
UKHW012300110422
401413UK00004B/1081